Disclaimer

The information included in this book is designed to provide helpful information on the subjects discussed. This book is not meant to be used to diagnose or treat any medical condition. For diagnosis or treatment of any medical problem, consult your own doctor. The author and publisher are not responsible for any specific health or allergy needs that may require medical supervision and are not liable for any damages or negative consequences from any application, action, treatment, or preparation, to anyone reading or following the information in this book. Links may change and any references included are provided for informational purposes only.

Anti-Inflammatory Diet

Heal Yourself
The Top 100 Best Recipes For
Chronic Inflammation

By Susan Hollister
Copyright © 2017

TABLE OF CONTENTS

INTRODUCTION 4

CHAPTER 1: CHRONIC INFLAMMATION 101 6

CHAPTER 2: PRO-INFLAMMATORY "BAD" FOODS 10

CHAPTER 3: ANTI-INFLAMMATORY "GOOD" FOODS 18

CHAPTER 4: INFLAMMATION REDUCERS 24

CHAPTER 5: CHRONIC INFLAMMATION ACTION PLAN .. 31

CHAPTER 6: BOUNTIFUL ANTI-INFLAMMATORY BREAKFAST RECIPES 35

CHAPTER 7: ANTI-INFLAMMATORY LUNCH RECIPES FOR HOME AND WORK 53

CHAPTER 8: DELICIOUS ANTI-INFLAMMATORY DINNER ENTREES 76

CHAPTER 9: SWEET AND SAVORY ANTI-INFLAMMATORY SNACKS 102

CHAPTER 10: SPECTACULAR ANTI-INFLAMMATORY SMOOTHIES AND JUICES 121

CONCLUSION 134

MY OTHER BOOKS 135

Introduction

I want to thank you and congratulate you for getting this book that contains proven steps and strategies to reduce and heal inflammation.

Chronic inflammation has become an epidemic. Just look at your friends and family. How many of them have diabetes, heart disease, arthritis, fibromyalgia or chronic pain? These are all caused by chronic inflammation. This book will help you manage and prevent chronic inflammation. In the chapters that follow, you will find activities, supplements, medications, and other solutions that will help you reverse your inflammation and alleviate its pain. You will discover foods to avoid and you will also learn which foods help to reduce inflammation.

Fighting chronic inflammation calls for lifestyle adjustments. The greatest changes you face will involve what you eat and drink. But don't panic; I promise you won't be stuck eating bland kale, nor are you doomed to eat the same few foods over and over again! No, you are about to enter into an adventure that will satisfy the food-lover in you while actively combating your inflammation. Prepare for a massive improvement in your quality of life.

I must admit, you will be exposed to some ingredients that are probably outside of your normal food repertoire. You'll be asked to cut back on or avoid certain foods, while eating more of others. To alleviate any anxiety you may be feeling right now, no, you don't have to do this all at once! You can go at your own pace, and when you start feeling better, you will naturally want to continue eating the foods that make you feel great.

You can take your time; begin to introduce one new food item each week. I've even removed the hassle of figuring out how to use these new ingredients; a large portion of this book consists of practical recipes designed to combat inflammation. I've provided plenty of recipes for each meal of the day as well as snacks, desserts, juices, and protein-packed smoothies.

As a chronic inflammation sufferer, you may find it necessary to give up a few foods you are hooked on, but these recipes will open up a whole new world of delicious flavors and textures, to satisfy the most demanding palate. There are 100 recipes here, enough to provide good eating and wonderful variety for months of culinary enjoyment.

Anti-inflammatory diets are anything but boring! They include fruits, vegetables, spices, herbs, yummy fats and tasty sweets. They are delicious! The best thing: they are easy to make. A few of the ingredients will call for a trip to a health food store, but most can be purchased at your local grocery store without making a dent in your budget.

The anti-inflammatory diet is the ultimate healthy lifestyle. In addition to healing your inflammation, it will also boost your immune system. Diabetics on this diet often find they don't need as much medication as they did before. You will probably notice greater energy and mental alertness, and you just might lose some weight in the process.

In addition to dietary adjustments, this book offers practical suggestions that can help soothe chronic inflammation. Explore inflammation-reducers such as meditation, yoga, herbal supplements, vitamins, minerals, sleep therapy, and sun therapy. To combine all these practical tips, I will help you develop your personal customized action plan to set you on the road to better health.

But first, let's discuss what we mean when we talk about inflammation. Next stop: Chronic Inflammation 101!

Chapter 1: Chronic Inflammation 101

Chronic inflammation is often referred to as a modern-day epidemic. It can trigger a variety of common diseases, among them diabetes, arthritis, heart disease, depression, and even cancer. In many cases, inflammation is induced by how we live; the modern lifestyle embraces – often without knowing it – deadly toxins and other inflammatory agents. If you suffer from chronic inflammation, you know what I'm talking about.

The good news is that chronic inflammation can be controlled, managed, and in many cases, totally reversed.

Chronic inflammation and acute inflammation are two very different things. Acute inflammation arises as the result of a traumatic event, such as a fall, a car accident or an illness. It is temporary, with little long-lasting impact on the body. Chronic inflammation, on the other hand, is a long-term condition that is far from temporary. It develops over a long period of time and causes great damage throughout the body.

To understand chronic inflammation, you must first understand how the immune system works. Our immune system keeps the body safe from diseases that would otherwise do great harm. When illness strikes, the bone marrow deploys white blood cells to the site of the infection to kill the invaders, after which the healing process can begin. Chronic inflammation can be triggered by a false alarm; a message goes out to deploy white blood cells, but there is nothing for them to attack.

When there is no real invasion for the white blood cells to combat, they don't know what to do and just hang out in the area waiting for the enemy to appear. The human body is not designed to accommodate loose white blood cells hanging out for an extended time. Eventually the cells get "bored" and start attacking normal, healthy cells. This opens the door for serious diseases to invade the body.

Diseases Caused by Chronic Inflammation

The list of diseases triggered by chronic inflammation is long. Almost every serious life-altering, disease can trace its beginning back to chronic inflammation. High on the list are:

- Cancers.
- Heart/cardiovascular disease.
- Diabetes.
- Depression.
- Allergies.
- Rheumatoid arthritis.
- Osteoporosis.
- Obesity.
- Pancreatitis.
- Stroke.
- Kidney disease.
- Respiratory diseases.
- Crone's disease.
- Alzheimer's disease.
- Age-related macular degeneration.

- Irritable bowel syndrome.

- Chronic fatigue.

- Fibromyalgia.

- Celiac disease.

- Autoimmune diseases.

You can easily see why chronic inflammation is considered an epidemic; it causes so many of our modern-day illnesses.

Symptoms of Chronic Inflammation

Depending on the type and location of the white cell attacks, an individual could experience one or more of the following symptoms:

- Depression.

- Long-term stomach issues.

- Inflamed bowel or signs of irritable bowel, including cramping, diarrhea and pain when evacuating.

- Swelling, redness, loss of function, and inadequate physical warmth to a part of the body.

- Intense tiredness.

- Pain.

- Breathing problems.

These are just a few of the symptoms associated with chronic inflammation.

Chronic Inflammation Triggers

Certain conditions and environmental factors can trigger inflammation and cause it to become chronic. Common triggers include:

Anxiety – Stress often allows inflammation to take hold in the body. The same parts of the brain that detect pain are the ones that activate white blood cells because of anxiety or stress.

Bad Air – Pollution, in the form of industrial pollutants, or even tobacco smoke, can do many bad things to the body. Breathing the stuff can trigger diabetes and can contribute to insulin resistance.

Sleep Deprivation – Lack of sleep can be a source of anxiety. Normal sleep patterns keep the body at an even keel, but any disruption can trigger the start of inflammation.

Menopause – White blood cells are affected by estrogen. Estrogen imbalance can mess with the formation of white cells

Age – As we grow older, the enzymes and hormones that keep white blood cells in check can become sluggish. This sluggishness can result in inflammation.

Diet – What you eat and drink can be the most influential inflammation trigger. Diets high in the wrong kind of fats just invite inflammation. However, you can use diet as a powerful tool to reverse it. A diet that avoids the wrong foods: bad fats and simple carbohydrates like sugar, can go a long way toward reducing, reversing, and preventing inflammation.

While we can't prevent aging, and some environmental triggers can be unavoidable, we can lessen their impact by making the most of the triggers we can easily control. One of the most effective ways of eliminating chronic inflammation from the body is through what you eat. The next few chapters of this book will explain what foods are bad — because they worsen the symptoms of chronic inflammation — and what will minimize the problem.

Chapter 2: Pro-Inflammatory "Bad" Foods

The most significant way to reduce the effects of chronic inflammation is to change your diet. About 70% of our immune cells reside in the digestive tract. Eating "bad" foods does increase instances of inflammation and strengthens the effects of the disease. The good news is, if you eat a healthy diet, you are already avoiding some of the "bad" foods, and will just need to tweak your diet here and there.

"Bad" foods include saturated fats, many dairy products, sugars, starches, and a few others in a category all their own. In this chapter, you will learn how these foods can wreak such havoc and exactly which edibles you need to avoid.

Saturated Fats

By now, everyone knows that saturated fats are not good for your body, but the danger is doubled for individuals with chronic inflammation. First, saturated fats easily add weight, one of the primary triggers for inflammation. Secondly, several studies have concluded that a high intake of saturated fats prevents substances in white blood cells from telling them to go dormant. Too much saturated fat keeps the white cells revved up in search-and-destroy mode instead of standing down in recognition that there is no longer any danger present.

I recommend limiting your saturated fat intake to a mere 10% of your daily calorie limit. If you are a meat eater, limit your meat intake to 1 meal per week. Marinate your meat in herbs, spices or unsweetened fruit juice before cooking.

Even more important, avoid trans fats. These are foods labeled as hydrogenated or partially hydrogenated oils. They include vegetable shortening, margarine, crackers, cookies, etc. Vegetable and seed oils may be processed with chemicals and should be avoided. Oils to avoid are soy, corn, sunflower, saffron and palm oils.

Processed foods are also considered "bad" foods, because they are frequently filled with chemicals that are "foreign" to your body. This would include protein bars, whipped spreads and even hot dogs. They are also present in pasteurized, dried, smoked, and grilled foods.

Fried foods are usually high in unhealthy fats, making them very bad for individuals with chronic inflammation. Fried foods contain Advanced glycation end products (AGEs). AGEs are created by the high-temperature frying process and are a major contributor to inflammation. Of course, this includes french fries, fried chicken, and fish sticks (sorry).

Avoid grain-fed meat. These animals are fattened quickly without the benefit of natural grasses. And, on a humanitarian note, the animals are usually confined to small areas and are seldom allowed out to exercise or see the light of day. Another problem is that these "manufactured" animals are fed antibiotics, which we then consume in the process of eating them for dinner. Those antibiotics can hang out in our bodies and trigger all sorts of inflammation.

Dairy

Many people have allergies to dairy products; if you have a reaction to dairy, you probably are experiencing a form of chronic inflammation. Dairy products can also increase your blood sugar. Higher blood sugar contributes to chronic inflammation. The solution is to limit your intake of cheese, milk, and other dairy products. The exception is unsweetened yogurt, which is on the good food list. Although yogurt is a dairy product, it contains probiotics that help to reduce inflammation.

Sugar

Refined sugar makes the body sluggish and it can wreak havoc on your immune system. When your antibodies come out to fight a problem, they have trouble going away because they just don't care anymore. Excessive glucose in your system slows down your digestive system, which prevents the white blood cells from getting enough energy to kill germs.

Sugar can make you susceptible to infections. You more easily come down with colds, the flu and other bugs. It also makes you more susceptible to cancer. Sugar raises blood sugar levels and contributes to obesity. For these reasons, it is best to avoid anything high in refined sugar content, such as baked goods, soft drinks, and definitely anything with high fructose corn syrup on the ingredients list.

This means you'll want to avoid snack bars, candy, coffee drinks, sweet tea, pies, cakes and all those really good tasting items. This doesn't mean you can't have any. Just cut way back, making them only a tiny percentage of everything you eat.

Starches

Starches can include anything made with flour, especially if it's refined. The refining process for flour strips the grain of valuable nutrients. This "refinement" also makes it harder for your body to digest these foods, by putting them in a form that is harder for your body to convert to fuel. The process can spike blood sugar, which in turn prompts your pancreas to dump large amounts of insulin into your system, taxing both your pancreas and your circulatory system. Starches include white rice, barley, rye, wheat, and products like pretzels, flour tortillas, cereals, and breads.

Vegetables like corn, peas, and potatoes are also considered starches. You have probably heard of people with celiac disease or gluten intolerance. These are just another form of chronic inflammation.

Miscellaneous

Some "bad" foods don't fit into any of these categories but still need to be avoided.

Nuts, especially peanuts, are a bad allergen. As the peanut grows underground, it can be affected by mold and fungus. These are often the actual cause of the allergic reaction and resulting chronic inflammation.

Commercial spice seasoning mixes, such as taco mix, contain artificial colors and preservatives that can trigger chronic inflammation. The chemicals in the coloring agents disrupt hormone function and increase the possibility of chronic inflammation. Dry salad mixes present the same problem.

Synthetic sweeteners can increase glucose intolerance and boost levels of bad bacteria in the system. Throughout this book, the one sweetener that will be recommended is stevia. This natural sweetening agent comes from the leaf of the stevia plant. You use stevia powder in the exact same proportion as sugar.

Alcohol morphs into sugar almost immediately upon consumption and can slow down your metabolism. It also contains bacteria that pass through into the intestinal lining where many of our immune cells reside.

Of course, this is only a partial list of foods that contribute to inflammation. I have compiled a summary list of the major offenders so you can see them at a glance. Don't worry; it's not all that bad. Just wait until you see the good foods!

You will find that almost everything on this "bad food" list is something you already know is bad for you. Also, just because a food is on this list, it does <u>not</u> mean you have to eliminate it from your diet entirely. **Moderation is the key.** For example, take vegetable oil. It's more healthy to use coconut oil instead, but if you *must* use vegetable oil on occasion, it's no major crime.

At-A-Glance "Bad" Food List

Fats and Proteins

- Fried foods including chicken, fish, and french fries.
- Any fast food including burgers and wraps.
- Egg rolls (fried).
- Hot dogs.
- Bacon.
- Margarine.
- Vegetable shortening.
- Red meat.
- Pork.
- Sausage.
- Cold cuts.
- Jerky.
- Whipped spreads.
- Vegetable, soy, corn, sunflower, saffron or palm oil.
- Pizza.
- Spice mixes.

Starches

- Bagels.
- Bread.

- Breakfast cereal (except for old fashioned rolled oats).
- Cornstarch.
- Cornbread or muffins.
- Crackers.
- Croissants.
- Doughnuts.
- Flour.
- Granola.
- Muffins.
- Noodles.
- Pancakes.
- Waffles.
- Pita bread.
- White rice.
- Taco and tortilla shells.

Sugars

- Candy.
- Cake.
- Cookies.

- Corn syrup.
- Honey.
- Jams and jellies.
- Molasses.
- Pastries.
- Pie.
- Pudding.
- Soda.
- Sugar.
- Artificial sweeteners.

Dairy

- Whole milk.
- Cheese except for parmesan, romano, and feta.
- Cottage cheese.
- Ice cream or other frozen treats containing milk.
- Mayonnaise.

Miscellaneous

- Fruit juice (heating process kills beneficial enzymes).
- Popcorn.

- Peanuts.
- Chips.
- Pretzels.
- Corn chips.
- Rice cakes.
- Spice mixes.
- Coffee drinks.

Try to avoid these foods as much as possible. One by one, you can replace them with the healthy foods you will find in the next chapter.

Chapter 3: Anti-Inflammatory "Good" Foods

If you already eat a fairly healthy diet, you will have no trouble incorporating these foods into your meals. In fact, you may already be enjoying them and just need a few tweaks to increase their presence in your meal planning. Some of the good foods that prevent and reduce chronic inflammation are as follows:

Omega 3 Fatty Acids

Omega 3 fatty acids are found in fish and fish oil. They calm the white blood cells and help them realize there is no danger, so they will return to dormancy. Wild salmon and other fish are good sources; I recommend eating them at least three times a week. Other foods rich in Omega 3s are flax meal and dry beans such as navy beans, kidney beans, and soybeans. An Omega3 supplement may be helpful, if you are not able to ingest enough of these foods.

Fruits And Vegetables

Most fruits and vegetables are anti-inflammatory. They are naturally rich in antioxidants, carotenoids, lycopene, and magnesium. Dark green leafy vegetables and colorful fruits and berries do much to inhibit white blood cell activity.

At least nine servings of fruits and vegetables each day is recommended. One serving is about a half-cup of cooked fruits and vegetables or a full cup if raw. The Mediterranean Diet, rich in fruits and vegetables, is often suggested to individuals suffering from chronic inflammation.

Protective Oils And Fats

Yes, there are a few oils and fats that are actually good for the chronic inflammation sufferer. They include coconut oil and extra virgin olive oil. Butter or cream is also fine to consume. Ghee, made from butter, is even better because it has the lactose and casein removed – the very ingredients that cause so much trouble if you have lactose intolerance or wheat sensitivity.

Fiber

Fiber keeps waste moving through the body. Since the vast majority of our immune cells reside in the intestines, it is important to keep your gut happy. Eat at least 25 grams of fiber every day in the form of fresh vegetables, fruits, and whole grains. If that doesn't provide enough fiber, feel free to take a fiber supplement.

Miscellaneous

Flavor your food with spices and herbs instead of bad fats and unsafe oils. Spices like turmeric, cumin, cloves, ginger, and cinnamon can enhance the calming of white blood cells. Herbs like fennel, rosemary, sage, and thyme also aid in reducing inflammation while adding delicious new flavors to your food.

Fermented foods like sauerkraut, buttermilk, yogurt, and kimchi contain helpful bacteria that tend to prevent inflammation.

Healthy snacks would include a limited amount of unsweetened, plain yogurt with fruit mixed in, celery, carrots, pistachios, almonds, walnuts, and other fruits and vegetables.

At A Glance "Good" Food List

Omega 3 Fatty Acids and Other Meats

- Wild salmon.

- Tuna.

- Herring.

- Halibut.
- Trout.
- Mackerel.
- Cod.
- Sardines.
- Snapper.
- Striped bass.
- Whitefish.
- Duck and goose.
- Turkey and chicken white meat.
- Flank steak.
- Sirloin steak.
- Prime rib.
- Game meat.
- Eggs (free range).
- Flax meal.
- Dry beans.

Fruits

- Strawberries.

- Blueberries.
- Cantaloupe.
- Grapefruit.
- Pineapple.
- Apple.
- Tomatoes.
- Avocado.
- Kiwi.
- Papaya.
- Raspberry.
- Lemon.
- Lime.
- Orange.
- Peaches.

Vegetables

- Broccoli.
- Onions.
- Cabbage.
- Carrots.

- Spinach.
- Sweet potatoes.
- Collard greens.
- Bell peppers.
- Bok choy.
- Brussel sprouts.
- Cauliflower.
- Chard.
- Green beans.
- Kale .
- Leeks.
- Olives

Protective Fats

- Extra virgin olive oil (opt for organic, if possible).
- Coconut oil.
- Organic butter.
- Almond oil.
- Avocado oil.

Fiber

- Almonds.

- Walnuts.

- Hazelnuts.

- Cashews.

- Macadamia nuts.

- Sunflower seeds.

- Brazil nuts.

Of course, this is not an exhaustive list. If a food is healthy, that is, if it does not contain bad oils, dairy, sweeteners, or other modifiers, consider it for your diet. Generally, the closer a food is to its natural state, the more nutritious it will be.

Chapter 4: Inflammation Reducers

Triggers for chronic inflammation can be suppressed by many different lifestyle choices. Here are a few other activities and materials that can help appease your white blood cells so they don't just hang around, attacking anything they find.

Activities

Meditation – Just five minutes a day of meditation can be beneficial if you suffer from chronic inflammation. It can reduce your stress levels and balance your emotions, thereby lowering white blood cell activity. Although there are no conclusive studies on this subject, the people I know who participate in meditation are generally very healthy.

Yoga – Yoga is a form of stretching and strengthening exercise that can facilitate your healing and help you become tuned in to your body's needs. Yoga can massage and stimulate internal organs more effectively than almost any other form of therapy. It helps to flush toxins from the body and to optimize the functioning of every organ and system.

Exercise – It is generally believed that people who participate in at least two hours of exercise each week have fewer inflammation flare-ups. This may be due to the endorphin release and stress level reduction caused by exercise. There's no need to go to extremes to experience the benefits. Simply walking for 20 minutes a day, four days a week, can significantly reduce your autoimmune sensitivity.

Sleep – Sleep deprivation is a common trigger for chronic inflammation. Your body needs a minimum of seven hours of uninterrupted sleep daily. This is critical, because your body uses this "down time" to provide healing and restoration in ways that can't be accomplished when you are awake. The best way to protect your health and fight inflammation is to get enough sleep each night.

Get Enough Sun – Sun exposure is how our bodies receive what we need to create vitamin D, a crucial element in combating inflammation. Deficiencies in vitamin D can enhance inflammation. If you're fair-skinned, the recommended dosage is 10 minutes of direct sunshine, taken outside when the sun is high, wearing a tank top and shorts, and no sunscreen. The darker your skin, the longer it takes to absorb enough sun for your body to generate enough vitamin D. Likewise, if it's too cool for a tank top and shorts, you won't absorb as much unless you spend more time in the sun.

Stay Away from Antibiotics, Antacids, and NSAIDS – These items destroy beneficial microorganisms in our gut that help to digest our food. When these organisms are killed, the intestinal wall is weakened and toxins are released into the system, activating white blood cells.

If you have to take antibiotics, double or triple the amount of probiotics you get daily. You can use probiotic pills, but I also recommend filling up on kefir and sauerkraut and taking at least five drops of oil of oregano each day. These will not prevent antibiotics from killing the harmful bacteria but they will replace the population of healthy bacteria indiscriminately killed by the antibiotic.

Stay Away from Airborne Toxins – By this I mean the whole range of toxins, from industrial pollutants to home pollution – primarily cigarette smoke. Some people are highly sensitive to chemical cleaning solutions. Regardless of your sensitivity level, you would do well to start exchanging these toxic solutions for less toxic (and less expensive) alternatives. Common household ingredients like vinegar, baking soda, and salt can do the job every bit as effectively as commercial cleaning solutions, but without exposing you to toxic chemicals.

Other Ingestibles Besides Food

Drugs – Here are several drugs commonly used in the treatment of chronic inflammation:

- Pentoxifylline enhances circulation to the brain and the extremities and inhibits white blood cells.

- Metformin is a diabetes drug that reduces inflammation.

- Low dose statin drugs are often used to reduce chronic inflammation. They block receptors of white blood cells by controlling cholesterol levels.

- Corticosteroids also reduce inflammation by controlling the action of white blood cells.

Supplements – Vitamins, minerals, enzymes and herbs can help control chronic inflammation:

- Fish oil gives the body those all-important omega 3 fatty acids that stop inflammation.

- Quercetin, also known as bioflavonoids, is a yellow plant pigment. It stabilizes the cells that release histamines, thus stopping allergic reactions, which are a form of inflammation. You can find quercetin as a dietary supplement. It also occurs naturally in apples, citrus fruit, berries, tomatoes, cruciferous vegetables (like broccoli, sprouts, and cabbage), and leafy greens.

- Bromelain is an enzyme that reduces inflammation. It is found primarily in pineapples. This enzyme is especially useful for sinus inflammations and it can reduce swelling from osteoarthritis.

- Curcumin, known as the "solid gold" of India, is a powerful anti-inflammatory found in the turmeric root. It can reduce inflammation in the eyes, help to calm down eczema, treat asthma, and even lessen food allergies. It also has antimicrobial properties that can kill molds, bacteria, and viruses and has even been known to kill certain cancer cells.

To benefit from this powerful substance, include at least two tablespoons of turmeric powder in your foods every day. If you can find the root itself, all the better; just grate the fresh root into your favorite dishes. Turmeric is a common ingredient in curry, so if you like curry, just add extra turmeric and you're good to go.

[handwritten note: 2 tablespoons tumeric every day]

You can easily add more turmeric into your life by sprinkling it on salads and adding it to soups and vegetables. The flavor is mild enough to use almost anywhere. It even makes a nice cup of hot tea.

- **Resveratrol** is a substance that appears in its highest concentration in the skin of grapes (which is carried forward, in lesser amounts, into red wine) and in the Japanese knotweed plant. It appears, in much lower concentrations, in blueberries, peanuts, pistachios, and cocoa. Resveratrol is absorbed in the mouth, so take your time when you eat your grapes.

  Resveratrol has been found useful when given to type 2 diabetics. It is considered an anti-inflammatory, but studies so far regarding resveratrol's effect on other inflammations have been inconclusive.

- **Flaxseed oil** is another great source for those wonderful omega 3s we've been talking about. It .is used to treat Crohn's disease, lupus, heart disease, colitis, and to benefit hair, skin, and nails.

- **Ginger** is a root that has been used for centuries to treat inflammations in the gastrointestinal tract. The active property, gingerol, has been found effective in treating nausea, seasickness, and morning sickness as well as reducing the swelling and inflammation of osteoarthritis and rheumatoid arthritis. It can also inhibit the growth of colorectal cancer cells and will kill ovarian cancer cells outright. All you need to treat an upset stomach is about a half-inch piece of ginger root, steeped in a cup of hot water.

There are numerous ways to add ginger to your diet. Any spicy food can be enhanced by the addition of ginger, whether in the form of ground spice or minced pieces of the fresh root. Add ginger to fruits and fruit drinks; sprinkle it on salads and meat dishes to provide an extra kick of intense flavor.

- Alpha lipoic acid is an antioxidant generated by your body. You can also get more by eating spinach or red meat. It helps the inflammation in diabetics and is especially effective in reducing neuropathy and aiding in the metabolism of glucose. Most healthy bodies generate enough of the substance, but supplements are available for those who need it.

- Selenium is a trace mineral that is found in organ meats and seafood. It serves as to inhibit the growth of inflammation. A normal, healthy diet will supply all the selenium your body needs.

- Zinc is a mineral found primarily in meat, but it is available in smaller amounts in peanuts, almonds, turnips, peas, and oats. Zinc is an antioxidant and is anti-inflammatory in nature. It serves as a general immunity booster that reduces inflammation and speeds healing.

Vitamins are also instrumental in keeping inflammation to a minimum or stopping it all together.

- A – Vitamin A helps to prevent inflammation and may help slow the progressions of arthritis. Beta-carotene is found in orange and dark brown fruits and vegetables, such as carrots, cantaloupe, sweet potatoes, spinach, and kale.

- B – Vitamins B6, B9 (folate), and B12 are helpful in controlling chronic inflammation. They reduce levels of homocysteine, a protein associated with heart disease and rheumatoid arthritis. B6 and B9 occur together in nuts, beans, peas, fruits and vegetables. B6 and B12 are found together in red meat, fish, and poultry.

- C – Vitamin C contains antioxidants that rid the body of the free radicals that damage cells. There is clinical evidence that vitamin C is just as effective in reducing inflammation as statin drugs, which are often much more expensive.

- D – We've already talked about the importance of getting enough sun exposure each day, in order for your body to produce enough vitamin D. You can also ingest vitamin D via fatty fish and egg yolks, but there is no conclusive evidence that taking a supplement will help with chronic inflammation. It is still better to get enough sunlight during the day.

- E – Vitamin E is known to help the skin, but it also helps heart issues and might help with Alzheimer's disease. In supplement form it is known as alpha-tocopherol. The best natural sources are sunflower seeds, almonds, spinach, kale, and plant oils. A half cup of almonds or sunflower seeds will satisfy your daily requirement for vitamin E.

- K – Vitamin K lowers inflammation and is found in all those lovely green vegetables we have available to us in the grocery store.

Diet is probably the most effective way to fight chronic inflammation. Staying away from pro-inflammatory foods and focusing on the ones that have anti-inflammatory properties is probably the best way to go about stopping or preventing inflammation. However, combined with healthy activity, a diet full of these recommended substances will go a long way toward restoring your health and reducing inflammation.

Chapter 5: Chronic Inflammation Action Plan

Making up an action plan to help yourself conquer chronic inflammation will get you off the couch and away from the refrigerator so that you can get better. What follows is a simple action plan without too much detail. You can personalize it, adding specifics that fit your own preferences and needs

Your action plan will begin with a purpose and a personal goal statement that clarify specifically what you are working to accomplish. along with a time limit on when to start and end the activity. It should state the resources you have available to you. Then you will include possible barriers to achieving the goal. Only when you've completed these items will you be prepared to spell out the step-by-step process of reaching your goal.

Chronic Inflammation Sample Action Plan

PURPOSE: To reduce chronic inflammation using several methods including diet, exercise, supplements and massage to eventually, resolve the problem.

GOAL STATEMENT: I will examine all resources available to me in order to choose the best methods to reduce and ultimately eliminate my own inflammation; I will develop meal menus and activities that I will start using within the next two weeks.

RESOURCES:

- Anti-Inflammatory and pro-inflammatory food lists, researched online

- Recipes for breakfast, lunch, dinner and snacks, researched online

- Exercises that will help to stop inflammation, found online, in books, or through my gym.

- Specific nutritional supplements that will reduce my inflammation, researched online and through the advice of doctor, chiropractor, nutritionist.

- Massage and other methods of physical therapy to treat chronic inflammation, researched online and via advice of doctor and other healthcare professionals.

BARRIERS:

- Limited money to purchase pro-inflammatory foods, purchase supplements or get a massage.

- I do not like to pack my lunch and would rather go out to eat.

- Limited time for food preparation.

- Physical limitations that prevent me from standing for a long time.

STEP BY STEP PLAN

1. Find anti-inflammatory recipes suitable for my needs. I will need enough for at least seven breakfasts, seven lunches, seven dinners, and 14 snacks.

2. Use these recipes to devise a meal plan for a week. .

3. Clean out the refrigerator and pantry, removing all pro-inflammatory foods.

4. Go shopping for anti-inflammatory foods.

5. Visit my physician and chiropractor for advice on supplements and exercises.

6. Purchase supplements and place them where you will see them and be reminded to take them regularly.

7. Start walking for 10 minutes a day, four days a week. Each week increase the length of the walk until you are walking for at least 20 minutes a day, four days a week.

8. Plan out other exercises and physical activities, schedule them and create reminders on your phone or on a physical chart. Plan a small reward you will enjoy after each time you exercise.

9. Set up regular appointments with a massage therapist skilled in treating chronic inflammation; schedule massages for at least once every other week.

When you walk, take your phone and a small notebook along with you; use these to record interesting things you see along the way, ideas you want to remember, and to-do items you don't want to forget. Take pictures along the way and write down observations you make while you are on the walk. I have even picked flowers growing wild along my path, dried them and placed them in my book. These activities ward off boredom and encourage you to experience life as a whole person – body, mind, and spirit. If you prefer to frequent a gym for targeted exercise, especially if the weather is contrary, you can use the time to focus your awareness on each part of your body and to interact with the people around you.

Notice how the food issues come first in this plan. They are the easiest to address and will have the greatest noticeable impact on your chronic inflammation. Review the information in Chapters 3 and 4 to ensure you are receiving the appropriate balance of the different nutrients.

Use the recipes in the chapters that follow to complete your weekly meal plans. You will find breakfast, lunch, dinner, snacks, smoothies and juices in the pages that follow, all designed to help you reduce inflammation, The best thing about these recipes is that they can be mixed and matched to make up just about any meal. Let's start with breakfast.

Chapter 6: Bountiful Anti-Inflammatory Breakfast Recipes

Start your day off right with a hearty breakfast that will leave chronic inflammation out in the cold. Eat oatmeal, eggs, fruit, and other good stuff that will keep you going without causing your white blood cells to run amok. Some of these recipes contain yogurt, because you need the probiotics offered by yogurt, but only in moderate amounts, to avoid excessive caloric intake. Even though I've warned you against non-cultured dairy products, some of these recipes include milk. However, the quantities are small and you can easily substitute alternatives like almond milk, coconut milk, or rice milk.

TASTE-OF-FALL OATMEAL

This oatmeal recipe contains wonderful spices and delicious maple syrup you can indulge in all year round. Oatmeal is a grain, but steel-cut or old-fashioned rolled oats are anti-inflammatory in nature.

Ingredients:

4 cups water
1/4 teaspoon ground ginger
1/4 teaspoon ground allspice
1 teaspoon ground cloves
1 1/4 teaspoon ground cinnamon
1/4 teaspoon ground coriander
1/4 teaspoon ground cardamom
1 cup steel-cut or old-fashioned oats
Maple syrup to taste

Directions:

- Pour water in a saucepan and bring to a boil. In a small bowl, combine all the spices.

- Once water boils, pour in the oats and the spices and cook as per package directions.

- When done, serve oatmeal in bowls, drizzled with maple syrup.

Yield: 4 servings

TROPICAL OATMEAL

Coconut and cacao add a tropical flair to this old standby. Cacao – unlike its highly processed cousin, cocoa – is chock-full of healthy nutrients.

Ingredients:

1 1/2 cups steel-cut or old-fashioned oats
3 to 4 cups of coconut milk
4 tablespoons chia seeds
3 tablespoons raw cacao (found at health food stores)
1 pinch of stevia for sweetening
1 cup frozen cherries, thawed
1 tablespoon dark chocolate shavings, or more
1 tablespoon coconut shavings (optional)
Maple syrup to taste

Directions:

- In a medium pan, over medium heat, bring the oats, coconut milk, chia, cacao and stevia to a boil.

- Lower the heat and simmer until oats are tender.

- Serve in bowls and top with cherries, chocolate, coconut shavings (optional), then drizzle with maple syrup.

Yield: 4 servings

APPLE PIE OATMEAL

This oatmeal treat tastes a little like apple pie and makes for a great start to your day.

Ingredients:

4 cups water
2 teaspoons pumpkin pie spice
1 cup steel-cut or old-fashioned oats
3/4 cup applesauce
2 tablespoons toasted pecans, ground
1 teaspoon stevia or more to taste
3 teaspoons extra virgin olive oil

Directions:

- Bring the water to boil in a medium saucepan over high heat. Stir in the pumpkin pie spice and oats and boil for 5 minutes, stirring so the mixture does not stick to the bottom of the pan.

- Turn heat down to simmer for 30 minutes.

- Add the applesauce, pecans, and stevia; mix well.

- Spoon into four bowls and drizzle with olive oil.

Yield: 4 servings

FRUIT-FILLED OATMEAL

You make most of this recipe the night before and poke it in the refrigerator to rest overnight. Pull it out in the morning and finish for a filling and delicious breakfast.

Ingredients:

1 1/3 cup low-fat cottage cheese
2 cups fat-free Greek yogurt

4 teaspoons extra virgin olive oil
4 teaspoons vanilla
3/4 cup steel-cut or old-fashioned oats
2 1/2 cups frozen chopped peaches, thawed
2 cups frozen blueberries, thawed
6 tablespoons slivered or chopped almonds
1/4 teaspoon allspice

Directions:

- In a bowl, combine the cottage cheese, yogurt, olive oil, and vanilla.

- Cover with plastic wrap and put in the refrigerator overnight.

- In the morning, cook the oats per package instructions.

- When done add the cottage cheese mixture and mix well.

- Top with fruit and allspice.

Yield: four servings

OPEN-FACED EGG SANDWICH

Eggs are a wonderful source of protein. The best-tasting eggs are laid by free-range chickens. Ghee is a form of butter, but without the lactose and casein that are allergens for many people. It is rich in vitamins A, D, and E and helps the body remove toxins.

Ingredients:

1/2 avocado
1 egg
1 slice of gluten-free toast
1 1/2 teaspoon ghee
1/4 c spinach leaves
Red pepper flakes to taste

Directions:

Smash the avocado and make it into a paste.

Scramble the egg.

Top the toast with the ghee and then spread on the avocado paste.

Top the toast with spinach leaves and then the scrambled egg.

Sprinkle some red pepper flakes on top and enjoy.

Yield: 1 serving

BAKED EGG AND VEGGIE CASSEROLE

This casserole uses some ham, but you can leave it out if you prefer. Ham is not inflammatory when eaten in moderation. The recipe does call for cream cheese, but if you prefer, you can easily find dairy-free cream cheese at a health food store. Use either eggs or egg substitute.

Ingredients:

1 teaspoon salt
6 roma tomatoes, peeled and chopped
1 teaspoon extra virgin olive oil
1/2 cup onions, finely chopped
2 tablespoon vegetable stock
1/2 cup chopped ham
1 cup spinach, chopped
5 eggs or 1 1/4 cups egg substitute
1/4 cup cream cheese
1/4 cup fresh chives, chopped
3 tablespoons plain almond milk

Directions:

- Preheat the oven to 350 degrees Fahrenheit and boil a kettle of water that will fit into a baking pan. Use 4 to 6 ramekins and spray with nonstick spray.

- Place the salt and tomatoes in a small bowl and toss. Spoon equal amounts into each of the ramekins.

- Add the olive oil to a skillet, add the onions, and cook about 1 minute. Add the vegetable stock and cook until the onions become translucent. Add the ham and warm through. Turn off the heat and add the spinach, tossing and allowing it to wilt ever so slightly.

- Whisk the eggs in a medium bowl and add the softened cream cheese, most of the chives (save some for garnish) and the almond milk. Pour this mixture over the tomatoes and spoon the skillet mixture on top.

- Set the ramekins in the baking pan and place in the oven a rack set in the middle. Carefully pour boiling water into the bottom of the pan until it is half way up the sides of the ramekins. Bake for 25 to 30 minutes. Remove the ramekins with tongs to serve immediately.

Yield: 4 to 6 servings depending on the size of the ramekins.

HARD-BOILED FRUITY BREAKFAST

At first glance, you may question the sanity of combining hard-boiled eggs with fruit, but it truly tastes delicious. This recipe will get you going in the morning and will sustain your energy until lunch. You can hard boil your eggs the night before. .

Ingredients:

6 egg whites from hard-boiled eggs
1 cup fresh or frozen and drained strawberries
1 apple, peeled and sliced

2 tablespoons raw almonds
1 tablespoon freshly grated ginger root
1 teaspoon extra virgin olive oil

Directions:

- Place the ingredients in a food processor or blender and process until chunky.

- Pour in chilled glasses and drink or spoon out this delectable morsel.

Yield: 2 servings

SMOKED SALMON EGG BREAKFAST

You won't need smoked salmon for this recipe; the smoky flavor comes from chipotle powder, and liquid smoke flavoring. It certainly fooled *my* taste buds!

Ingredients:

6 eggs or 1 1/2 cups egg substitute
1/2 teaspoon ground turmeric
1/2 teaspoon dry mustard
1/2 teaspoon ground chipotle powder
1/2 teaspoon liquid smoke flavoring
1 (7–ounce) can of salmon, drained
2 1/2 teaspoons extra virgin olive oil

Directions:

- In a bowl, whisk the eggs, turmeric, dry mustard, chipotle powder, and liquid smoke. In another bowl, flake the salmon and set it aside.

- Heat the oil in a skillet over medium heat. Wait until the pan is hot, then add the egg mixture and sprinkle the flaked salmon on top.

- Do not scramble, but gently lift up the cooked sides and allow the uncooked eggs to run underneath.

- When no longer runny, slide the eggs out onto a plate, then and flip the eggs upside down back into the skillet and cook until done. Cut in wedges and serve with some cooked asparagus or broccoli.

Yield: 4 servings

BREAKFAST EGG TART

This recipe uses mozzarella cheese and you can find this cheese made with skim milk in most grocery stores. It is less likely to add to any inflammation.

Ingredients:

1/2 cups onion, finely chopped
1 (14.5–ounce) can of diced tomatoes, drained
18 green or black pitted olives, rinsed, drained and chopped
1 cup skim Mozzarella cheese, shredded
6 eggs or 1 1/2 cups egg substitute
1 1/2 teaspoons extra virgin olive oil
1 teaspoon basil
1 teaspoon dill
1/2 teaspoon pepper
1/4 teaspoon salt

Directions:

- Preheat the oven to 350 degrees, Fahrenheit.

- Grease an ovenproof skillet, add half of the onions and half of the tomatoes, and then sauté for about 2 minutes.

- Turn off the heat and stir in the olives and mozzarella.

- Place the rest of the onions and tomatoes in a blender along with the eggs, olive oil, herbs, salt, and pepper; blend until smooth.

- Pour into the skillet and transfer the skillet to the preheated oven. Bake for 25 to 30 minutes. The mixture will puff up and turn a golden brown.

- Serve with a fruit salad.

Yield: about 4 servings

WHICH-CAME-FIRST BREAKFAST SKILLET

You tell me, was it the chicken or the egg? In this recipe at least, the egg wins out, but not by much. You're looking at one hearty breakfast that'll give you a real protein boost.

Ingredients:

1 cup onions, finely chopped
1 pound frozen broccoli, thawed
1/4 cup water
1/4 cup skim or 2% milk
4 eggs or 1 cup egg substitute
2 teaspoons extra virgin olive oil
3 tablespoons pesto
1/4 cup low-fat cottage cheese
Salt and pepper to taste
1 large cooked chicken breast, finely shredded
3 cloves minced garlic
1/4 cup sun-dried tomatoes (optional)

Directions:

- Place the onions in a skillet with the frozen broccoli. Add the water and cover cooking over medium for about 5 minutes. After making sure the broccoli is cooked through, remove from heat and drain.

- In a bowl whisk together the milk, eggs, olive oil, pesto, cottage cheese, salt, and pepper.

- Stir in the chicken, garlic, and optional tomatoes.

- Pour the mixture into a greased skillet. Cover and cook over medium heat until the eggs set on one side. Flip this "tart" and cook on the other side.

Yield: 4 servings

ITALIAN EGGS

This breakfast is delicious, with plenty of vegetables and even some Garbanzo beans for extra protein.

Ingredients:
1 teaspoon extra virgin olive oil
1/4 cup green bell pepper, diced
1/4 cup white onion, diced
1/4 cup canned garbanzo beans, rinsed, drained and lightly mashed
2 eggs or 1/2 cup egg substitute
1/4 teaspoon basil
1/4 teaspoon oregano
Salt and pepper to taste
1 ounce low-fat provolone cheese
1/2 cup salsa

Directions:

- Heat a skillet on the stove and after it becomes hot, add the olive oil. Pour in the peppers and onions and sauté until soft. Add garbanzo beans and heat through.

- In a bowl combine the eggs and herbs. Pour over the top of the vegetables and make sure the egg mixture covers the bottom of the pan.

- Add the provolone cheese and cover the skillet. Cook on low until the eggs are set and the cheese has melted. Season with salt and pepper.

- Fold the cooked eggs onto a plate and top with salsa.

Yield: 2 servings

EGG AND VEGGIE WRAP

Flour tortillas are pro-inflammatory, but corn tortillas are usually gluten free. They will work if you can't find gluten-free flour tortillas. Make this 'to go' breakfast whenever you are on the run.

Ingredients:

2 tablespoons red onion, chopped
2 tablespoons green bell pepper, chopped
3 eggs or 3/4 cup egg substitute
1 (10-inch) gluten-free tortilla

Directions:

- Spray a small skillet with non-stick spray and place over medium heat. Sauté the pepper and onion in the skillet until softened.

- Add the egg and scramble until done.

- Place the scrambled eggs on the tortilla and roll it up.

Yield: 1 serving

Apple Banana Breakfast Cupcakes

This recipe is both gluten- and dairy-free. It contains both oatmeal and quinoa, giving you a double dose of anti-inflammatories.

Ingredients:

Olive oil
3/4 cup water
1/2 cup dry quinoa
1/2 cup applesauce
1 cup mashed banana
1/2 cup almond milk
1/4 cup honey
1 teaspoon vanilla
2 1/2 cups dry old-fashioned oats
1 teaspoon cinnamon
1 apple, peeled, cored and chopped into chunks
1 banana, sliced

Directions:

- Preheat the oven to 375 degrees Fahrenheit and grease a muffin tin with olive oil.

- Pour the water into a medium pan and bring it to a boil. Add the dry quinoa and reduce to a simmer for about 12 minutes. Fluff and measure out 1 cup. Let the quinoa cool completely and dry out.

- In a bowl, mix the applesauce, mashed banana, almond milk, honey, and vanilla.

- In another bowl, mix the dry oatmeal and cinnamon. Gradually add this to the liquid ingredients, mixing in thoroughly.

- Stir in the cooled quinoa and apple chunks.

- Fill muffin tins to the top and add a slice or two of the banana to each muffin. Bake 20 to 25 minutes and let cook about 5 minutes before serving warm. They are also delicious cold, if any of the muffins last that long.

Yield: 12 cupcakes.

SPICY QUINOA BOWL

Here's more luscious quinoa, this time in a bowl with spices and nuts along with a few blueberries to sweeten the deal. The chia seeds at the end are optional but it does give the dish a nice crunch.

Ingredients:
2 cups cooked and cooled quinoa
1 cup thick cashew milk
1/4 teaspoon ground cinnamon
1/8 teaspoon ground nutmeg
1/4 teaspoon ground ginger
1 tablespoon toasted walnuts, cashews or pecans
1 cup fresh or frozen blueberries
1 1/2 teaspoon honey
1 teaspoon chia seeds (optional)

Directions:

- In a medium saucepan, combine the quinoa with the cashew milk. Warm over medium-low heat.

- Add the spices, nuts and blueberries and heat through.

- Spoon into 2 bowls, drizzle with honey, and sprinkle with chia seeds.

Yield: 2 servings

LEMON QUINOA WITH CHIA SEEDS AND ALMONDS

This dish is almost like lemon pudding, but with the added crunch of chia seeds and almonds.

Ingredients:
1 cup quinoa

4 1/2 tablespoons maple syrup or honey
1 1/2 cups almond milk
1 tablespoon chia seeds
3 tablespoons slivered almonds
1/4 teaspoon sea salt
1/4 teaspoon lemon zest

Directions:

- Cook the quinoa per package instructions.

- Remove from heat and set aside for about 5 minutes.

- Fluff the quinoa with a fork, then add the remaining ingredients.

- Mix well and serve warm.

Yield: 4 servings

STRAWBERRY QUINOA

Use either fresh or frozen strawberries for this breakfast treat, which is super-easy to make. If you desire a little extra sweetness, mix in a teaspoon of stevia with the strawberries.

Ingredients:

1 serving of quinoa, cooked per package instructions
1 cup strawberries, sliced if fresh
1/2 tablespoon maple syrup
1/4 cup chopped cashews

Directions:

- Place the quinoa in your breakfast bowl.

- Mix in the strawberries and maple syrup. Sprinkle with cashews.

- Pick up your spoon and dig in.

Yield: 1 serving

ZESTY COCONUT BASMATI RICE PUDDING

Basmati rice is better for inflammation than regular white rice. If you would rather use brown rice, you will just need to cook it a little longer.

Ingredients:

1 cup water
1 (13.6-fluid ounce) can coconut milk
1 cup long grain basmati rice
3/4 cup orange juice, fresh squeezed
2 teaspoons vanilla
1/8 teaspoon sea salt
1 teaspoon ground cinnamon
1 teaspoon ground ginger
1 tablespoon orange zest
3 tablespoons maple syrup

Directions:

- Combine the water, coconut milk, rice, orange juice, vanilla and salt in a medium saucepan and bring to a boil.

- Reduce to a simmer and cover, but leave ajar for steam to escape. Cook for 30 minutes or until liquid is absorbed.

- Stir in the spices, zest, and syrup. Mix well.

- Serve warm or cold.

Yield: 4 servings

CITRUS-APRICOT BREAKFAST SALAD

This will wake you up in the morning with a citrus fresh flavor.

Ingredients:
2 grapefruit, peeled, pith removed, and sectioned
2 oranges, peeled and sectioned
4 apricots or 2 peaches, skin and stone removed and sliced
1 tablespoon honey

Directions:

- Place segments of citrus fruit and slices of apricot or peaches in a large bowl.

- Stir in the honey and enjoy.

Yield: 2 servings

HONEY-LIME BREAKFAST SALAD

Talk about flavor. Use any fruit you like to make this delicious salad. If you prefer to omit the mint, it will taste different, but still fresh.

Ingredients:
1 cup dry quinoa, rinsed
2 cups water
1 1/2 cups chopped fruit
1/3 cup fresh mint leaves, chopped
1 lime
2 tablespoons honey
A dash of salt
1/4 cup mint leaves for garnish

Directions:

- Toast the dry quinoa in a heated saucepan over medium heat for 1 minute.

- Pour in the water and bring the pan to a boil.

- Reduce to a simmer, cover, and cook for 15 minutes.

- Remove from the heat and let sit for 5 minutes. Once cool, put in a bowl, cover with plastic wrap and place in refrigerator overnight.

- In the morning, mix the fruit into the quinoa and add the chopped mint leaves.

- In a small bowl whisk the lime juice, honey, and salt, then pour over the quinoa mixture. Garnish with mint.

Yield: 4 to 6 servings

GINGER-LEMON BREAKFAST SALAD

Make this salad the night before so it is nice and chilled for in the morning.

Ingredients:
1 tablespoon squeezed lemon juice (1/2 lemon)
1 tablespoon fresh ginger root, grated
1 pear, sliced
2 kiwis, sliced
1 cup frozen pitted cherries, thawed

Directions:

- Mix all ingredients in a serving bowl.

- Refrigerate and let it chill overnight.

- In the morning, your fruit salad is ready to serve.

Yield: 4 servings

Some of these breakfast recipes are just as easy and delicious to use for lunch. The breakfast salads could easily serve as an after-dinner dessert. And speaking of lunch, it's about that time, so let's move on to explore some imaginative noontime fare.

Chapter 7: Anti-Inflammatory Lunch Recipes for Home and Work

Many of the following recipes are easily packaged and taken to work. Not only do they make a delicious addition to your family's culinary repertoire, you can serve them to guests as well.

KALE CAESAR SALAD

This salad is great all by itself, but you can also roll it in a tortilla to make a delicious wrap. Feel free to swap vegetables to suit your preference.

Ingredients:

1/2 coddled egg (See instructions below.)
1 clove garlic, minced
1/2 teaspoon Dijon mustard
1/8 cup fresh-squeezed lemon juice
1 teaspoon honey
1/8 cup extra virgin olive oil
Salt and pepper to taste
6 cups curly kale
3/4 cup shredded skim Parmesan cheese
1 cup raw broccoli florets
1/4 cup sliced almonds

Directions:

<u>To coddle an egg</u>

A coddled egg is just a slightly cooked egg that has a runny consistency.

- Take an egg out of the refrigerator about 30 minutes prior to using; you want it at room temperature.

- Boil water in the teakettle and prepare an ice bath for the egg by putting ice in a bowl and adding water.

- Set the uncracked egg gently in a large mug. Pour the boiling water over the egg and let it sit for exactly one minute. Remove the egg immediately and submerge it in the ice bath for two minutes before using.

To mix the dressing

- Mix the coddled egg, garlic, mustard, lemon juice, and honey in a small bowl by whisking vigorously.

- Add the olive oil, salt, and pepper to taste; whisk well.

To combine the salad

- Place the kale, Parmesan cheese, and broccoli in a large bowl.

- Pour the dressing over top and toss.

- Sprinkle almonds over top and serve.

Yield: 2 servings

CHICKEN KALE WRAP

This is similar to the previous recipe, but it is served as a wrap. If you prefer, you can serve this without the wrap, as a salad. It's very tasty either way.

Ingredients:

1/2 coddled egg (See instructions below.)
1 clove garlic, minced
1/2 teaspoon Dijon mustard
1/8 cup fresh squeezed lemon juice
1 teaspoon honey

1/8 cup extra virgin olive oil
Salt and pepper to taste
4 cups curly kale
3/4 cup shredded skim Parmesan cheese
1 cup cherry tomatoes, quartered
1 baked chicken breast, shredded

To coddle an egg

A coddled egg is just a slightly cooked egg that has a runny consistency.

- Take an egg out of the refrigerator about 30 minutes prior to using; you want it at room temperature.

- Boil water in the teakettle and prepare an ice bath for the egg by putting ice in a bowl and adding water.

- Set the uncracked egg gently in a large mug. Pour the boiling water over the egg and let it sit for exactly one minute. Remove the egg immediately and submerge it in the ice bath for two minutes before using.

To mix the dressing

- Mix the coddled egg, garlic, mustard, lemon juice, and honey in a small bowl by whisking vigorously.

- Add the olive oil, salt, and pepper to taste; whisk well.

To combine the salad

- Place the kale, Parmesan cheese, cherry tomatoes and chicken in a large bowl.

- Pour the dressing over top and toss.

- Spread the mixture over two whole-wheat flatbreads or tortillas and roll them up.

Yield: 2 servings

BEET SALAD

Beets are a powerful antioxidant, so this recipe, chock-full of delicious, healthy ingredients, can easily become a frequent visitor at your table. You can easily multiply this recipe to serve a large group of people.

Ingredients:

1 large raw beet, grated coarsely
1 large apple, cored and diced
1 large carrot, peeled and grated
1 tablespoon chopped almonds
2 tablespoons fresh squeezed lemon juice
2 tablespoons fresh parsley, chopped
2 tablespoons flaxseed oil or extra virgin olive oil
2 cloves garlic, minced
4 cups mixed greens
Salt and pepper to taste

Directions:

- In a medium-sized bowl, combine the beets, apple, carrot and almonds.

- In a smaller bowl, mix together the lemon juice, parsley, oil, and garlic. Whisk well and pour over the beet mixture.

- Place the greens in a large bowl and mix in the lemon juice mixture, tossing well.

- Divide the greens among 4 plates and top with the beet mixture.

Yield: 4 servings

AVOCADO SPINACH SALAD

Either make your own humus or purchase some at the store to make this salad.

Ingredients:

2 cups baby spinach
1 handful alfalfa sprouts
1/2 avocado, thinly sliced
1/2 orange bell pepper, diced
1/2 carrot, grated
2 tablespoons prepared hummus
1 tablespoon extra-virgin olive oil

Directions:

- Combine the spinach, sprouts, avocado, bell pepper and carrot in a serving bowl.

- In a small bowl whisk the hummus and olive oil. Pour this over the veggies, tossing well.

Yield: 2 servings

BROCCOLI APPLE SALAD WITH CRANBERRIES OR RAISINS

This sweet salad with yogurt is a favorite in my house. I've never seen a healthy salad be requested at potluck dinners more frequently than this one.

Ingredients:

3 apples, cored and diced (leave the skin on)
4 cups fresh broccoli florets
1/2 cup sunflower seeds or slivered almonds
1/2 cup dried cranberries or raisins

1/4 cup red onion, minced
2 tablespoons Dijon mustard
1/4 cup honey
1 cup plain yogurt

Directions:

- In large serving bowl combine the first five ingredients.

- In another bowl, mix the mustard, honey, and yogurt and whisk until thoroughly combined.

- Pour over the salad and toss well.

- Chill for 30 minutes before serving

Yield: 6 servings

TUNA SALAD, REVISITED

This is nothing like your grandmother's tuna salad. It contains a variety of fresh flavors that blend well together and are anti-inflammatory, to boot! I've included several ingredient options you can swap out to suit your taste; feel free to experiment.

Ingredients:

1 (2.5-ounce) can of water-packed tuna, drained well
1/4 cup chopped Kalamata olives (Option: use your favorite olive)
2 tablespoons red onion or shallots, minced fine
2 tablespoons fire-roasted red peppers, chopped
2 tablespoons fresh basil leaves, finely chopped
1 tablespoon fresh-squeezed lemon juice
1/4 cup mayonnaise or creamed avocado
Salt and pepper to taste
2 romaine lettuce leaves

Directions:

- Put the tuna, olives, onion, peppers, and basil into a large bowl.

- In a small bowl, combine the mayonnaise with the lemon juice. When it is well-mixed, pour over the salad and mix well.

- Place the romaine leaves on 2 plates and scoop out the tuna salad with an ice cream scoop, placing the ball atop the lettuce.

Yield: 2 servings

TROPICAL QUINOA SALAD

Quinoa is very nutritious and filling. This dish will prove an attractive addition to your salad repertoire.

Ingredients:

1 cup quinoa, rinsed well
2 cups water
1 cup apple, cored and finely chopped
1/2 red onion, peeled and finely chopped
2 tablespoons honey
Juice of 1 lime
1 tablespoon extra virgin olive oil
1 large mango, chopped
1/4 cup cilantro, finely chopped
1/4 cup mint, finely chopped
1/2 inch piece of ginger root, peeled and finely chopped
1/2 teaspoon sea salt
1 avocado, chopped
1 cup chopped cashews
3 cups romaine lettuce, roughly chopped

Directions:

- Boil the water and add the quinoa to cook. Simmer covered 15 to 20 minutes.

- Set aside to let cool. You can do this ahead of time or spread the hot quinoa out so that it cools well and dries a bit.

- Combine the onion and apple in a large serving bowl.

- In a smaller bowl, whisk the honey, lime juice, and olive oil together. Add to the onion apple mixture. Then, add the quinoa and mango, tossing everything well.

- Add in the cilantro, mint, and ginger; toss lightly. Season to taste with salt and pepper.

- Divide the romaine lettuce on 4 plates and scoop the salad on top.

- Garnish with avocado and sprinkle with cashews.

Yield: 4 servings

CURRY-GINGER QUINOA SALAD

This salad is warmly spiced with a combination of delicious flavors.

Ingredients:

1 cup well drained quinoa
1/2 teaspoon grated ginger root
1 teaspoon curry powder
2 cups water
1 tablespoon apple cider vinegar
1/8 cup extra virgin olive oil
1/2 teaspoon of additional curry powder
1/8 teaspoon salt
1/4 cup walnuts

1/4 cup fresh parsley, chopped
1/2 cup shelled edamame

Directions:

- Heat a skillet and toast the quinoa for about 1 minute.

- Add the ginger and 1 teaspoon curry; mix over medium heat for another minute or so.

- Add the water and bring the mixture to a boil. Turn down the heat and simmer until the water is absorbed, about 10 minutes.

- In a small bowl combine the vinegar, olive oil, 1/2 teaspoon curry and salt; whisk together until well-combined.

- Place the walnuts, parsley, and edamame in a large bowl, then add the cooked quinoa. Pour the dressing over top and mix well.

Yield: 2 large servings

QUINOA SALAD WITH GREEN TAHINI DRESSING

The roasted parsnips and carrots give this salad a lovely flavor. I like to serve this in the winter because of the roasted root vegetables.

Ingredients:

2 medium parsnips, peeled and cut into 1/2-inch pieces
2 medium carrots, peeled and cut into 1/2-inch pieces
1 small yellow onion, halved and thinly sliced
1 tablespoon extra virgin olive oil or coconut oil
1/4 teaspoon sea salt
4 to 5 sprigs of fresh thyme
2 cups water

1 cup red quinoa
Salt and pepper to taste
1 cup tahini
1/2 cup freshly squeezed lemon juice
1/4 cup extra virgin olive oil
1 cup fresh parsley, chopped
1 tablespoon fresh dill, chopped
3 scallions, thinly sliced
2 cloves garlic, crushed
1/8 teaspoon salt
A pinch of red pepper flakes
Water, if needed.

Directions:

- Cover a baking sheet with parchment paper and top with parsnips, carrots and onion, . Drizzle with olive oil and sea salt. Toss until evenly coated and make sure the vegetables do not overlap.

- Cover with thyme sprigs and roast in a preheated 425 degree oven for 25 to 30 minutes, stirring halfway through. The vegetables should look caramelized.

- While roasting the vegetables, put the water on to boil and add the quinoa. Cover, reduce to a simmer, and cook for 15 minutes or until the liquid is absorbed. Season with salt and pepper to taste.

- Place the tahini, lemon juice, olive oil, parsley, dill, scallions, garlic, salt, and red pepper flakes in a blender. Blend until creamy, adding water as necessary to maintain the consistency.

- After the vegetables are cooked, toss them in the pot with the quinoa and mix well. Transfer to a platter and drizzle with the tahini dressing.

- This dressing keeps well in the refrigerator for several weeks, if it isn't consumed immediately.

Yield: 4 servings

CITRUS SALAD

Anyone who likes citrus fruit will *love* this salad. It is surprisingly filling with a little sweet-and-sour action to wake up your taste buds.

Ingredients:

2 large tangerines, peeled
1 pink grapefruit, peeled
3 navel oranges, peeled
1/2 cup dried cranberries, plus additional for garnish
1/4 teaspoon ground cinnamon
2 tablespoons honey
2/3 cup crystallized ginger, minced
1 (16- to 17.6-ounce) container of plain Greek yogurt
1/4 cup brown sugar

Directions:

- Separate all the citrus fruit into segments and cut the large segments into bite-sized morsels. Place in a serving bowl along with any juice from the fruit.

- Add the dried cranberries, cinnamon, and honey. Cover and chill 1 hour or overnight.

- Mix the crystallized ginger into the yogurt and spoon it over the fruit.

- Sprinkle with brown sugar and dried cranberries, then serve.

Yield: 4 servings

PAD THAI IN THE RAW

This recipe is full of vegetables and has some spiciness to it.

Ingredients:

1 large carrot, peeled
1 medium zucchini that has skin removed
1/2 cup shredded purple cabbage
1/2 cup cauliflower florets
1/4 cup mung bean sprouts
1 large green onion, chopped
1 tablespoon fresh squeezed lime or lemon juice
2 tablespoons wheat free tamari
1 tablespoon honey
2 tablespoons tahini
1/4 teaspoon garlic, peeled and minced
1/2 teaspoon peeled ginger root, grated

Directions:

- Make vegetable noodles by using a vegetable peeler to cut thin strips of the carrot and zucchini. Place the vegetable "noodles" in a large serving bowl along with the cabbage, sprouts and onion.

- Whisk together the remaining ingredients in another bowl. The mixture will be very thick, but will thin out when mixed with the vegetables. Pour the sauce over the vegetables and toss well.

- Cover the bowl with plastic and let it marinate a few hours; marinate overnight for even better flavor.

Yield: 2 servings

SPANISH FRITTATA

This egg dish is perfect for lunch as it is a little more substantial than breakfast frittatas.

Ingredients:

1/2 cup coconut milk
12 large eggs
1/4 teaspoon sea salt
2 tablespoons coconut or extra virgin olive oil
1 clove garlic, minced
1 small red onion, peeled and chopped
1/2 cup green bell pepper, chopped
1/2 cup mushrooms, sautéed in coconut or olive oil
1 cup fresh spinach

Directions:

- Preheat the oven to 375 degrees Fahrenheit.

- Whisk the coconut milk and eggs with the salt and set aside.

- Place the oil in a large ovenproof skillet and heat. Add the garlic, onion, and bell pepper, sautéing until the onions become translucent.

- Add the mushrooms and heat through.

- Add the spinach and mix while letting it wilt.

- Remove from heat, place vegetables in a bowl and set aside.

- Turn heat to low and add a little more oil if necessary. Whisk the eggs in a bowl and add to the skillet.

- As it cooks, lift the edges with a spatula and let the liquid part of the eggs fall underneath. Keep cooking until the edges are not runny and the middle is somewhat set.

- Place the vegetables in the center of the eggs.

- Place the skillet into the oven and cook about 5 minutes until the eggs are completely set and light brown.

- Slide half of the frittata onto a plate and flip it back into the skillet, with the uncooked side down.

- Stick the skillet back in the oven for 5 more minutes. Serve immediately.

Yield: 2 servings

CUSTOMIZED OMELET

You can put just about anything in an omelet. Try any kind of vegetable, any cheese, cottage cheese, and almost any meat. The mouthwatering savoriness of your omelet comes from the herbs and spices you use. I've chosen Herbes de Provence, a tantalizing mixture of seasonings from the Provence region of France, as an example, but you can substitute almost any mix of spices. This is the perfect recipe for experimenting with different flavors; be bold in your spice and herb mixing and you can hardly go wrong!

Ingredients:

1/2 to 1 cup sautéed vegetables (cabbage, peppers, carrots, mushrooms, etc)
1 tablespoon coconut oil or organic butter
6 eggs
1/4 cup sweet onion, peeled and chopped fine
Salt and pepper to taste
1 teaspoon Herbes de Province
1 slice Swiss cheese or 1/4 cup low fat cottage cheese

Directions:

- Grease a skillet. Peel and slice all vegetables and sauté until softened. Set aside.

- Add the oil or butter to the pan. Toss in the onion and sauté until translucent.

- In a small bowl whisk the eggs, salt, pepper, and herbs. Pour this mixture in the pan over the onions.

- Use a spatula to lift the edges of the omelet and let the runny part of the egg flow underneath. Once most of the egg is cooked, slide the omelet out onto a large plate. Flip the omelet back into the skillet to cook the other side until the eggs are set.

- Place the cheese and reserved vegetables on one half of the omelet and fold the other half over to sandwich in the cheese and vegetables.

- Cover the skillet and cook on low heat for about 2 minutes or until heated through. If your pan is ovenproof, set it in a 350-degree oven for 5 to 8 minutes. Serve immediately.

Yield: 2 to 3 servings

SPINACH CUPCAKES

Enjoy this delicious and nutritious lunch item with fresh fruit. Do not use Parmesan from a can because it is too dry; grate your own.

Ingredients:

12 ounces fresh spinach leaves
1/2 cup low-fat cottage cheese
1/2 cup Parmesan cheese, freshly grated
2 large eggs

1 clove of garlic, crushed
1/4 teaspoon salt
1/4 teaspoon pepper
1/4 teaspoon red pepper flakes

Directions:

- Preheat the oven to 400 degrees Fahrenheit.

- Pulse the spinach in batches in a food processer to a fine chop, then place in a mixing bowl.

- Add the remaining ingredients and stir with a wooden spoon to mix well.

- Grease an 8-muffin tin and fill each depression to the top with the spinach mixture.

- Bake for 20 minutes or until lightly brown and set. Grate a little additional Parmesan cheese over the top for added flavor.

Yield: 8 muffins.

CHICKEN AND WHITE BEAN CHILI

Eat this for lunch on a cold day; it'll warm you right up. You can use chicken broth instead of water if you prefer; just make sure it's a low salt broth.

Ingredients:

2 tablespoons extra virgin olive oil or coconut oil
1 pound boneless, skinless chicken breasts, cut into bite-sized pieces
1/2 teaspoon salt
1/4 teaspoon pepper
2 cloves garlic, diced
1 medium onion, peeled and diced

1 cup corn (tastiest when fresh from the cob)
1 (4-ounce) can green chilies, chopped
2 (15-ounce) cans great northern beans, drained
1/8 teaspoon cayenne pepper
2 teaspoons chili powder
1 teaspoon cumin
3 cups water

Directions:

- Grease a dutch oven well, then add the oil.

- Sprinkle the chicken breast pieces with salt and pepper and place in the dutch oven, browning both sides.

- Lower the heat and add garlic and onions to the pan, then cook until the onion is translucent.

- Add the corn, chilies, beans, cayenne, chili powder and cumin and mix well.

- Add the water and bring to a boil.

- Simmer uncovered for 1 hour.

- Dish out each serving and garnish with a little cheese and cilantro on top.

Yield: about 8 servings

SWEET POTATO WITH ROASTED RED PEPPER SOUP

This soup is creamy, delicious, and filling.

Ingredients:

2 tablespoon extra virgin olive oil
1 clove of garlic, minced
2 medium onions, peeled and chopped

1 (4-ounce) can diced green chilies
1 (12–ounce) jar roasted red peppers, drained and chopped, with liquid reserved.
1 teaspoon ground coriander
2 teaspoons ground cumin
1 teaspoon salt
3 to 4 cups sweet potatoes, peeled and cubed
4 cups vegetable broth
1 teaspoon lemon juice
2 tablespoons cilantro, minced
4 ounces non-dairy cream cheese, softened

Directions:

- In a dutch oven, heat the olive oil, then add the garlic and onion. Sauté until soft.

- Add the chilies, red peppers, coriander, cumin, and salt; cook for about 3 minutes.

- Stir in the reserved juice from the peppers as well as the broth, then add the sweet potatoes.

- Bring the pot to a boil, then reduce to a simmer and cover. Cook about 10 to 15 minutes or until the potatoes no longer hard.

- Stir in the lemon juice and cilantro and remove from the heat. Let the soup cool slightly.

- Place half of the soup in a blender along with the cream cheese. Blend until smooth, then return the processed soup to the pot and mix well.

- Heat through, stirring, before serving.

Yield: 6 servings

SPICY GINGER AND CARROT SOUP

This recipe comes from India so you know it is a bit on the spicy side. It will warm you up and even the kids will like it because it is sweet too.

Ingredients:

1/2 teaspoon yellow mustard seeds
1 teaspoon coriander seed
3 tablespoon almond or flax oil
1/2 teaspoon curry powder
1 tablespoon gingerroot, peeled and minced
1 1/2 pounds carrots, peeled and sliced into thin rounds (about 4 cups)
2 cups yellow onion, peeled and chopped
1 1/2 teaspoons grated lime peel
Salt and pepper to taste
5 1/2 cups vegetable or chicken broth (low-salt)
2 teaspoons lime juice
Garnish with plain yogurt

Directions:

- Grind the mustard and coriander seed to a fine powder in a spice mill.

- Heat the oil in a dutch oven, then add the powder along with the curry powder and cook about 1 minute.

- Add the ginger and cook for another minute, stirring constantly. Add the ginger, carrots and chopped onion, seasoning with salt and pepper. Cook until the onions are softened.

- Add 5 cups of broth and bring to a boil. Reduce to a simmer and cook uncovered until the carrots become tender, about 30 minutes.

- Cool the soup for 15 minutes.

- Work in batches to puree the soup in a blender or use an immersion blender until it is all smooth.

- Return the pureed soup to the pot and add 1/4 cup of broth, stirring to mix well. If it seems too thick, add a little more broth.

- Stir in the lime juice and heat through before serving. Add a dollop of yogurt atop each serving as garnish.

- This recipe reheats well, so feel free to make it up a day ahead.

Yield: 6 to 8 servings

TURMERIC VEGETABLE SOUP

Turmeric is good for chronic inflammation and this soup includes a big tablespoon of it!

Ingredients:

1 tablespoon extra virgin olive oil
1 onion, peeled and diced
2 stalks celery, finely chopped
1 medium carrot, peeled and finely chopped
2 teaspoons garlic, minced
1/2 teaspoon grated ginger root
1 tablespoon ground turmeric (or more as preferred)
1/4 teaspoon cayenne
3 to 4 cups water
1 (32-ounce) carton of vegetable broth
1 teaspoon salt
1/4 teaspoon pepper
3 cups cauliflower florets, chopped
1 bunch of kale, chopped
1 (15-ounce) can great northern beans, drained and rinsed

Directions:

- Warm the oil in a large dutch oven and add the onion.
- Cook until the onion softens and begins to brown.
- Add the celery and carrots and cook for 5 more minutes.
- Stir in the garlic, ginger, turmeric and cayenne, cooking for another minute.
- Add the water, broth, salt, and pepper. Bring to a boil, then reduce to a simmer.
- Add the cauliflower, cover and simmer for 15 minutes or until the cauliflower is tender.
- Add the kale and beans and cook until kale is wilted and the beans heated through.
- Serve piping hot.

Yield: 6 servings

CHICKEN AND SWEET POTATO SOUP

This sweet potato soup includes chickpeas and is very filling and delicious.

Ingredients:

1 tablespoon extra virgin olive oil
2 stalks of celery, diced
1 cup onion, peeled and diced
4 cups low-salt chicken broth
1 large red sweet potato peeled and diced
1 cup canned chickpeas
1/2 teaspoon dried thyme

1 1/2 cup cooked and chopped chicken breast

Directions:

- Heat the oil in a dutch oven and add the celery and onion.

- Cook until softened, about 5 minutes.

- Add the chicken broth and sweet potato, bring to a boil, and then reduce to a simmer

- Cook until the potato is tender, about 15 to 20 minutes.

- Stir in the chickpeas, thyme, and chicken breast. Heat through before serving.

Yield: about 4 servings

WHITE BEAN ROAST GARLIC SOUP

In this recipe, you roast the garlic in the oven and add it to the soup almost at the end of cooking. Roast garlic has a distinct flavor that makes this soup especially delectable.

Ingredients:

1 pound dry cannellini beans
4 cups low-salt chicken broth
4 cups water
4 fresh sage leaves
1 head of garlic with outer skin removed but the cloves left intact
2 teaspoons extra virgin olive oil
Kosher salt to taste

Directions:

- Place the dry beans, water and broth in a Crock-Pot and add the sage.

- Cover and cook on high for 4 hours or on low for 8 hours. Check halfway through to ensure the beans are getting soft.

- Preheat the oven to 400 degrees, Fahrenheit.

- Cut a square of aluminum foil about 7 by 7 inches square and place the peeled garlic head in the center. Drizzle with olive oil and salt, then pull the sides of the foil up and seal the garlic inside. Bake on a baking pan for 25 to 30 minutes. Remove from the oven and set aside to cool.

- Once the garlic has cooled, squeeze out all the cloves and put the resulting paste in a blender along with half of the soup.

- Blend until smooth, then return the soup mixture to the Crock-Pot and mix well.

- Add salt and pepper to taste before serving to the hungry masses.

Yield: 6 servings

Now that you have lunch under your belt, let's go on to dinner entrees.

Chapter 8: Delicious Anti-Inflammatory Dinner Entrees

Dinner should be the apex of your meals for the day, although with all the great anti-inflammatory recipes in this book, it may be hard to choose just one highlight. On an anti-inflammatory diet, you can eat beef in moderation, say, 2 red meat dishes in a week. To help balance your diet, here are some recipes for fish, chicken, beef, and vegetarian meals.

SALMON WITH ZUCCHINI

Several herbs are used in this recipe along with lemon to give it a well-rounded flavor that brings out the unique savor of salmon.

Ingredients:

2 tablespoons packed brown sugar
1 tablespoon Dijon mustard
2 cloves of garlic, minced
1/2 teaspoon dried oregano
1/2 teaspoon dried dill
1/4 teaspoon dried rosemary
1/4 teaspoon dried thyme
1/8 teaspoon kosher salt
Pinch of fresh black pepper
4 zucchini, chopped
2 tablespoons extra virgin olive oil
1/2 teaspoon sea salt
1/4 teaspoon black pepper
4 (5-ounce) salmon fillets
2 tablespoons fresh parsley, chopped fine (for garnish)

Directions:

- Preheat the oven to 400 degrees Fahrenheit, cover a baking pan with parchment paper and spray with non-stick spray.

- Whisk the brown sugar, mustard, garlic, oregano, dill, rosemary and thyme and add the 1/8 teaspoon salt and pinch of pepper. Set aside.

- Place the zucchini on the baking sheet in a single layer and drizzle with the olive oil and season with 1/2 teaspoon salt and 1/4 teaspoon pepper.

- Place the salmon atop the zucchini on the baking sheet. Brush well with the brown sugar-herb combination.

- Place in the oven and cook about 16 to 20 minutes or until the fish flakes easily using a fork. Garnish with parsley and serve.

Yield: 4 servings

SEARED SALMON ARUGULA

Arugula has a fresh and different flavor than spinach and it goes very well with the flavor of salmon.

Ingredients:

Salmon

1 1/2 tablespoons extra virgin olive oil
1 1/2 tablespoon fresh squeezed lemon juice
1/4 teaspoon Kosher salt
1/8 teaspoon ground pepper
2 center-cut salmon filets about 6 ounces each

Salad

3 cups baby arugula leaves
2/3 cup peeled and diced cucumber
1/4 cup red onion, peeled and thinly sliced
Salt and pepper to taste

1 tablespoon extra virgin olive oil
1 tablespoon red wine vinegar

Directions:

Salmon

- Place the olive oil, lemon juice, salt and pepper in a shallow bowl and whisk well. Add the salmon filets and coat well. Cover and let rest 15 minutes.

- Heat a nonstick skillet, oiled with butter-flavored spray.

- Cook the salmon with the skin side down for 2 to 3 minutes over medium high heat. Keep shaking the pan and lifting the salmon with a spatula so it does not burn.

- Turn down the heat to medium, cover the pan, and cook 4 more minutes or until fish is cooked through. The skin should be crisp and the meat should flake easily.

Salad

- In a serving bowl combine the arugula, cucumber, and onion; season with salt and pepper to taste.

- Whisk together the olive oil, and red wine vinegar, then pour over the salad, tossing lightly.

- Serve alongside the salmon.

Yield: 2 servings

PEACH-AND-LAVENDER-CHUTNEYED SALMON

If you don't like the flavor of lavender, use mint or basil. Apricots, nectarines or plums can take the place of peaches, if you prefer.

Ingredients:

1/2 cup dry white wine
1/2 cup water
2 pounds of salmon fillets, cut in 4 pieces
1/2 tablespoon coconut oil
1 1/2 teaspoon dried parsley
1 1/2 teaspoon garlic, minced
1/4 teaspoon salt
1 pinch pepper
1 large onion, peeled and minced
1 tablespoon minced garlic
1/4 teaspoon red pepper or chili flakes (optional)
2 pounds peaches, peeled, stoned and diced
Zest of 1 lemon
1/3 cup red wine vinegar
1/4 cup honey
1/2 teaspoon salt

Directions:

- Place wine and water in a large non-stick skillet and cook over medium high heat for about 5 minutes. It should not boil, but be a bit steamy.

- Add the salmon to the poaching liquid, dot it with coconut oil and add the parsley, garlic, salt, and pepper.

- Bring to a boil. Immediately reduce the heat to a barely simmering level. Poach until the flesh is firm, 10 to 15 minutes.

- To make the chutney, combine the onion, garlic, red pepper, peaches, lemon zest, vinegar, honey, and salt in a saucepan and bring to a boil.

- Boil for 15 minutes stirring occasionally. Mix in lavender and remove from heat. Let sit 5 minutes before using.

- Top the poached salmon with the chutney.

- You may have some chutney left over from this recipe. Just keep it in the refrigerator and use it on crackers or with another fish dish.

Yield: 4 servings

BAKED LEMON HALIBUT

Halibut has a mellower flavor than salmon, so it benefits from a spicy marinade. In this recipe, the halibut is marinated and then served with papaya salsa. This dish needs to marinate for 2 hours or overnight. This recipe contains a lot of ingredients, but your taste buds will agree that this dish is well worth your effort.

Ingredients:

1 cup papaya, cubed
1/4 cup red onion, peeled and chopped fine
1/4 cup red bell pepper, cubed
1 small jalapeño pepper, seeded and minced
1/2 cup fresh cilantro leaves
2 tablespoons fresh squeezed lime juice
1 tablespoon extra virgin olive oil
3 tablespoons fresh squeezed lemon juice
1 tablespoon grated ginger root
1/2 teaspoon ground pepper
1/2 cup more cilantro
1 tablespoon grated lemon zest
2/3 cup water
3 medium fennel bulbs, trimmed and sliced
9 black peppercorns
6 (6-ounce) halibut steaks, cut in half, lengthwise

Directions:

- To make the salsa, combine the papaya, onion, red pepper, jalapeño, cilantro, and lime juice in a small bowl. Smash it together with a fork until it turns into a chunky

- paste. Cover and place in the refrigerator until ready to serve.

- In another bowl, combine the olive oil, lemon juice, ginger, pepper, 1/2 cup more cilantro and lemon zest. This will be your marinade. Cover the bowl and let it chill in refrigerator for 2 hours.

- Place the fish in a non-stick greased baking pan and pour the lemon juice mixture over the top. Cover and refrigerate for 20 minutes.

- Preheat the oven to 400 degrees Fahrenheit. While oven preheats, place 2/3 cup of water in a saucepan, along with the sliced fennel and peppercorns. Cover and cook at a high temperature for 6 to 8 minutes or until the fennel is just becoming tender. Remove from heat.

- Bake the halibut in the marinade for 5 minutes. Remove from the oven, flip the halibut to the other side and bake for another 5 minutes. When done, it should flake easily with a fork.

- Drain the fennel and divide it among 6 plates. Lay the halibut steaks atop the fennel. Spoon about a tablespoon of papaya salsa over the fish and serve.

Yield: 6 servings

BAKED BASIL TROUT

Trout is enhanced by the basil in this flavorful recipe.

Ingredients:

2 teaspoons extra virgin olive oil
1/4 cup fresh squeezed lemon juice
1/4 cup fresh basil leaves, minced
4 (6-ounce) rainbow trout fillets

1/4 teaspoon salt
1/2 teaspoon ground black pepper
1 small lemon, thinly sliced

Directions:

- Preheat the oven to 350 degrees Fahrenheit. Combine the olive oil, lemon juice, and basil in a bowl and whisk to mix the sauce. Set aside.

- Grease a 9 by 13-inch baking pan. Place the fillets in the dish and sprinkle with salt and pepper. Top with thin lemon slices. Drizzle half of the basil sauce over top.

- Bake for 13 to 15 minutes or until the fish flakes easily with a fork. Drizzle the rest of the basil sauce over the top and serve.

Yield: 4 servings

FANCY SOLO SEA SCALLOPS

In this recipe, you bake the bay sea scallops in individual dishes. Use ramekins or other ovenproof dishes. Bay scallops are large, but you might want to double the recipe so each person gets two scallops.

Ingredients:
4 (3-ounce) bay scallops
1/4 cup white wine
1/4 cup old-fashioned rolled oats
1/4 cup fresh-squeezed lemon juice
1 teaspoon lemon pepper
2 tablespoons low-fat shredded cheddar cheese

Directions:

- Place the scallops in a shallow baking dish, cover, and marinate in the white wine overnight in the refrigerator. Turn them over a couple times during the evening.

- Preheat the oven to 350 degrees Fahrenheit.

- Drain the scallops and put into individual oiled dishes.

- Sprinkle with oats, drizzle with lemon juice, sprinkle with lemon pepper, and top with cheese.

- Bake for 10 to 15 minutes.

Yield: 4 servings

SESAME SHRIMP

Hemp seeds pack a lot of additional protein into this dish.

Ingredients:

2 teaspoons sesame oil
1/4 cup tamari sauce
2 tablespoons hemp seed
2 tablespoons coconut oil
1 pound large shrimp, peeled and deveined
1 medium orange pepper, seeded and sliced
1 small yellow summer squash or zucchini cut into matchsticks
1 small yellow onion, peeled and thinly sliced
3 ounces shitake mushrooms with the stems removed and thinly sliced
2 cloves garlic, minced
2 cups rainbow chard, roughly chopped
3 cups of cooked quinoa

Directions:

- Whisk together the sesame oil, tamari, honey, and hemp seed in a small bowl and set this sauce aside.

- Using a large non-stick skillet, heat the coconut oil and add the shrimp. Stir-fry over high heat for about 2 minutes or until pink. Place in a bowl and set aside.

- In the same skillet, add the orange pepper, squash, onion, and mushrooms; stir-fry for about 5 minutes. Add the garlic and stir-fry for another minute.

- Add the chard and cook until wilted, about 2 minutes.

- Add the sauce and simmer until it thickens slightly.

- Stir the shrimp back into the skillet and cook for 2 minutes.

- Serve over cooked quinoa.

- Option: swap out the shrimp for chicken and you'll have a delicious chicken sesame dish.

Yield: 4 servings

COCONUT CHICKEN

Chicken breast meat melts in your mouth in this flavorful recipe. The coconut enhances the natural flavor and the almond meal adds a hint of crunch.

Ingredients:

1 large egg
1 pressed garlic clove
1/4 teaspoon salt
3/4 cup almond meal
1/2 cup shredded, unsweetened coconut flakes
1 chicken breast, halved

Directions:

- Preheat the oven to 350 degrees Fahrenheit and line a baking sheet with parchment paper.

- Whisk the egg in a bowl and add the garlic and salt. Whisk well. Add the almond meal and stir into a paste. Place the coconut on a dinner plate.

- Dip the chicken into the egg mixture and coat it evenly. Roll each breast into the coconut until covered, then place on the baking sheet.

- Bake for 35 to 40 minutes, turning the breasts over after 25 minutes.

Yield: 2 servings

MUSHROOMED CHICKEN

I use baby bella mushrooms for this dish. They have a nuttier flavor than plain mushrooms, but you can use those, if you prefer. I recommend against canned mushrooms, however.

Ingredients:

2 (3-ounce) chicken breasts, halved
1/4 teaspoon salt
1/4 teaspoon pepper
2 tablespoons extra virgin olive oil
1 cup sweet onions, peeled and sliced
8 ounces fresh mushrooms, thinly sliced
Pinch of salt
10 ounces fresh baby spinach
1/2 cup water
1 tablespoon apple cider vinegar

Directions:

- Preheat the oven to 400 degrees Fahrenheit.

- Season the chicken on both sides with salt and pepper. Place the olive oil in an ovenproof skillet over medium high heat. Add the chicken and cook for about 5 minutes.

- Flip the chicken breasts over and cook for 2 minutes before adding the onions and mushrooms with another pinch of salt. Cook for another 5 minutes.

- Place the skillet in the oven and cook about 15 to 20 minutes. Meanwhile, steam the spinach.

- Remove the chicken from the skillet and set it aside.

- Place the skillet on the stove and crank up the heat. Pour in the water and stir up the brown bits. Cook until the water is reduced by half, about 2 minutes, then remove from heat.

- Spoon this sauce over the chicken and serve alongside vinegar-drizzled spinach.

Yield: 2 servings

GINGER CHICKEN

Ginger is one of the greatest anti-inflammatory spices. The ginger and sesame oil in this recipe give it a slight Asian hue.

Ingredients:

1 tablespoon sesame oil
1 tablespoon extra virgin olive oil
3 large or 4 small chicken breasts, cubed
1 1/2 cup yellow onion, peeled and thinly sliced
1 tablespoon garlic
2 cups snow peas
1 cup carrots, peeled and cut in flat vertical slices
4 cups broccoli florets, cut in bite-sized pieces
1 1/2 tablespoon freshly-grated ginger root

1/2 to 3/4 cup water
4 cups cooked rice

Directions:

- Use a wok or a large non-stick skillet. Heat both oils and add the cubed chicken.

- Sauté until browned and mostly cooked through (about 5 minutes).

- Add the onion, garlic, snow peas, carrots, broccoli and ginger. Stir-fry for 2 minutes and add the water. Add only 1/2 cup at first but if the mixture starts to dry out, add a little more, 1 tablespoon at a time.

- Stir and cook until the chicken is done, the vegetables are tender but still a little crisp, and the water is reduced to a glaze. This can take about 15 to 20 minutes.

- Serve over brown rice.

Yield: about 4 servings

HOITY-TOITY CHICKEN CASSEROLE

You wouldn't normally think of a casserole as anti-inflammatory, but this one uses almond meal, oatmeal, and almond milk, making it not only mouthwatering-good but good for you. The artichoke hearts add a touch of class to this otherwise mundane dish.

Ingredients:

1 (14–ounce) can artichoke hearts, drained and quartered
1 pound fresh green beans, trimmed and cut in 2 inch pieces
1 tablespoon extra virgin olive oil
2 minced cloves of garlic
2 1.2 tablespoons almond meal
1 3/4 cups almond milk

2 cups chopped, cooked chicken breast
Salt and pepper to taste
Cayenne pepper to taste
2/3 cup old-fashioned rolled oats
Butter-flavored cooking spray

Directions:

- Drain the artichoke hearts, quarter them, wrap in paper towels, and squeeze them dry. Set aside.

- Cook fresh green beans in a pot of boiling water for 4 to 6 minutes or until tender. Drain and set aside.

- Preheat the oven to 425 degrees Fahrenheit.

- Heat the olive oil in a saucepan over medium heat. Add the garlic and sauté about 1 minute.

- To make the roux, whisk in the almond meal, cooking for 1 minute while stirring to prevent it from browning. Gradually whisk in the almond milk and bring it to a boil.

- Reduce to a simmer and cook, stirring constantly, until the sauce thickens, about 3 minutes.

- Stir in the green beans, the cooked chicken, and the artichoke hearts. Season with salt, black pepper, and cayenne pepper before placing in a 2-quart baking dish.

- Spread the oats on a dinner plate and spray with the cooking oil until slightly moistened. Spread the oats atop the casserole, then take a large spoon and press the oats gently into the casserole, moistening them in the almond milk.

- Bake for 15 minutes or until the sauce begins to bubble.

Yield: about 4 servings

COLORFUL CRUNCHY CHICKEN

The crunch in this dish comes from the vegetables and the sliced almonds. Use any two colors of bell pepper. The vibrant colors in this dish even make it *taste* better!

Ingredients:

3 cups broccoli florets, steamed and softened
3 large or 4 small boneless, skinless chicken breasts, cooked and sliced
1 tablespoon extra virgin olive oil
1 red bell pepper, seeded and chopped
1 yellow bell pepper, seeded and chopped
1 cup red onion, peeled and chopped
1 zucchini, peeled and chopped
3 cloves of garlic, peeled and minced
1/4 cup sliced almonds
Salt and pepper to taste

Directions:

- Steam the broccoli.

- While it is steaming, heat the oil in a sauté pan over medium heat.

- Add the cooked chicken, peppers, onion, zucchini and garlic.

- Cook, stirring frequently until everything is cooked through and the vegetables are tender-crisp.

- Add the steamed broccoli and heat through.

- Place in serving bowl, top with the almonds, season with salt and pepper, and serve proudly.

This recipe serves 4.

STEAK MEDALLIONS WITH SPINACH

This recipe calls for an olive tapenade to be spread over the meat. If you don't like olives, substitute pesto or another type of thick sauce, as desired. This steak is grilled instead of baked.

Ingredients:

Tapenade

8 ounces Kalamata olives, pitted and minced
3 garlic cloves, minced
2 tablespoon fresh Italian parsley, minced
2 tablespoon capers, rinsed and drained
2 teaspoon lemon peel, minced
Black pepper, to taste
3 tablespoons extra virgin olive oil

Steak

1 pound flank steak
1/4 cup olive tapenade
3 cups fresh baby spinach (for stuffing)
3 cups fresh baby spinach (for garnish)
Kosher salt and black pepper to taste

Directions:

Tapenade

- In a small bowl, combine olives, garlic, parsley, capers, lemon peel, and black pepper, stirring until well-mixed.

- Add olive oil and mix thoroughly.

Steak

- Heat the grill to medium high.

- Set the flank steak in front of you with the grain running left to right. Trim off any excess fat, along with any loose stringy matter. Slightly square off the steak so that when it is rolled up, the rolls will be basically even.

- With a razor-sharp knife, work to make two thin slices that are connected on one end. Take your time and concentrate on keeping your knife horizontal to the countertop. Slicing with the grain, leave the two slices attached on the right end by about an inch. Open up the slices, creating a long rectangle of meat.

- Spread the tapenade over the steak and then lay the spinach leaves neatly on top. Leave about an inch on the right edge free, so the filling won't squeeze out when it is rolled up.

- Roll the steak into a log, and tie off with cooking twine every 2 inches.

- Season the steak with salt and pepper.

- Grill covered, turning the steak occasionally, for about 15 to 20 minutes.

- Let the meat rest for 5 minutes before slicing into medallions. To serve, place a few spinach leaves on a plate, then top with a beef slice.

Yield: about 6 slices

FAJITA SALAD

This salad calls for a delicious cilantro-lime dressing, which follows.

Ingredients:

1/4 cup extra virgin olive oil
Juice of 1 lime
2 cloves of garlic, minced
1 teaspoon oregano
1/2 teaspoon onion powder
1 teaspoon chili powder
1 teaspoon ground cumin
Salt and pepper to taste
2 pound flank steak
1 green bell pepper, seeded and thinly sliced
1 orange bell pepper, seeded and thinly sliced
1 red bell pepper, seeded and thinly sliced
1 sweet onion, peeled and thinly sliced
8 cups romaine lettuce, chopped
1 avocado, halved, peeled and thinly sliced

Directions:

- To make the marinade, whisk together the olive oil, lime juice, garlic, oregano, onion powder, chili powder, and cumin in a small bowl and season with salt and pepper to taste.

- Place the steak in a gallon-sized re-sealable bag and pour in the marinade. Close and let it set in the refrigerator for at least 30 minutes, turning the steak occasionally. If you wish, you can marinate the meat overnight.

- Drain the marinade and heat 1 tablespoon of extra virgin olive oil in a non-stick skillet over high heat. Cook the steak about 5 minutes per side for rare, longer to taste, for more well-done.

- Remove from heat and let the steak rest for at least 10 minutes. Cut thinly against the grain and set aside

- Add another tablespoon of olive oil to the skillet, then add the peppers and onion. Cook until the peppers are soft and the onion is translucent. When finished, they should be lightly caramelized. This should take about 10 minutes. Set aside.

- Place the romaine lettuce in a bowl, pour the peppers and onions over the lettuce, and add the avocado. Heat up the steak and add this to the salad.

- Serve with cilantro-lime dressing.

Yield: 6 servings

CILANTRO-LIME DRESSING

Any leftover dressing will keep, refrigerated, for about a week and a half.

1 cup cilantro, stems removed
2 tablespoons Greek yogurt or smashed avocado
1/2 cup non-dairy sour cream
2 cloves garlic, minced
Pinch of salt
Juice of 1 lime
1/4 cup extra virgin olive oil
2 tablespoons apple cider vinegar

Directions:

- Combine the cilantro, yogurt, sour cream, garlic, salt, and lime juice in a food processor.

- Mix the olive oil and vinegar and pour in a steady stream while processing.

Yield: about 2 cups of dressing

POMEGRANATE STEAK

To remove the seeds from a pomegranate easily, cut in half. Hold the half, seed down, over a large bowl; with a ruler or a knife, slap the back of the pomegranate. The gelatinous seeds should fall out into the bowl.

Substitute chicken or lamb in this recipe, if desired.

Ingredients:

1 teaspoon extra virgin olive oil
1 pound strip steak
1/2 teaspoon salt
1/4 teaspoon ground black pepper
1/2 cup pomegranate seeds (1 small pomegranate)
1 can chickpeas, drained
2 scallions, sliced
1 tablespoon fresh-squeezed lemon juice
1/4 cup fresh mint leaves
2 tablespoons extra virgin olive oil
1/4 teaspoon salt
1/4 teaspoon pepper
4 cups baby arugula

Directions:

- Set a skillet on the stove over medium heat and add a teaspoon of olive oil. Season the steak with 1/2 teaspoon salt and 1/4 teaspoon pepper, then cook it in the skillet to desired doneness. Let the steak rest on a cutting board for a few minutes before slicing.

- Combine the pomegranate seeds, chickpeas, scallions, lemon juice, mint leaves and 2 more tablespoons of the extra virgin olive oil in a large serving bowl.

- Season with 1/4 teaspoon of salt and pepper.

- Stir in the arugula and serve this salad alongside the steak slices.

Yield: 4 servings

GINGER-BEEF STIR-FRY

This recipe includes the anti-inflammatory turmeric and ginger along with a multitude of vegetables.

Ingredients:

2 tablespoons coconut oil
2 cloves garlic, minced
1 yellow onion, peeled and sliced
1/2 red bell pepper, seeded and thinly sliced
1 pound flank steak, cut into thin strips
2 tablespoon fresh squeezed lemon juice
2 teaspoons grated ginger root
1 teaspoon turmeric
2 tablespoons tahini
2 tablespoons wheat-free tamari
1 tablespoon apple cider vinegar
1 cup fresh green beans, tipped and cut in 1 inch pieces
2 cups fresh broccoli florets
1 cup snow peas sliced diagonally
Salt and pepper to taste
Brown rice

Directions:

- Place the coconut oil in a hot skillet over medium heat and melt.

- Stir in the garlic, onion and bell pepper and sauté for about 7 minutes.

- Add the beef and stir-fry for 5 to 7 minutes.

- Add the lemon juice, ginger, turmeric, tahini, and vinegar. Cook for about 1 minute.

- Add the beans, broccoli and snow peas and cook over medium heat another 15 minutes.

- Season with salt and pepper and serve over brown rice.

Yield: 4 servings

BOK CHOY STIR-FRY

This recipe is meatless but the combination of mushrooms, peppers, and a pile of bok choy make for a satisfying meal.

Ingredients:

2 cups shitake mushrooms, chopped with stems removed
2 red peppers seeded and cut into thin strips
6 cups bok choy, chopped into 2 inch pieces
1 tablespoon coconut oil
1 yellow onion, peeled and chopped
4 cloves of garlic, peeled and minced
1 tablespoon freshly-grated ginger root
2 teaspoons tamari sauce
1 teaspoon sesame oil
1 tablespoon fresh squeezed lemon juice
1/4 cup slivered or sliced almonds

Directions:

- Cut the mushrooms, peppers, and bok choy before beginning to cook.

- Use a dutch oven over medium-high heat and melt the coconut oil.

- Add the onion and stir-fry for 2 to 3 minutes or until it softens.

- Add the garlic and sauté for another minute.

- Stir in the mushrooms and ginger, then cook for 2 more minutes.

- Toss in the peppers and stir-fry for 2 minutes or until slightly softened.

- In a bowl whisk the tamari, sesame oil and lemon juice together. Pour it over the mixture in the pot and stir to combine all the ingredients.

- Add the bok choy, cover the pot and let it steam for 3 to 4 minutes.

Yield: 3 servings

RED LENTIL SQUASH CURRY

This stew is full of protein and hearty flavors. It is designed to warm you up; it's especially cheering in cold, blustery weather.

Ingredients:

1 teaspoon extra virgin olive oil
2 cloves garlic, minced
1 yellow onion, peeled and chopped
1 tablespoon curry powder (add more if you can take it)
1 cup red lentils
4 cups low-sodium vegetable broth
3 cups butternut squash, cooked and diced
1 cup collard greens
1/2 teaspoon salt
1/4 teaspoon black pepper
1 tablespoon freshly-grated ginger root

Directions:

- Put a dutch oven on the stove and heat the olive oil.

- Add the garlic and onion and cook over medium-low heat until the onion is translucent.

- Stir in the curry and cook for 2 minutes.

- Add the broth and lentils and bring to a boil. As soon as it reaches a rolling boil, lower the heat to a simmer and cook for 10 minutes, uncovered.

- Stir in the cooked squash and greens.

- Cover the pot and simmer over medium for about 5 minutes.

- Season with salt and pepper and add the ginger. Serve hot.

Yield: 4 servings

AFRICAN STEW

Enjoy the rich earthy flavor of this stew any time you want a hearty meal.

Ingredients:

1 cup great northern beans, soaked overnight and drained
1 tablespoon coconut oil
2 cloves garlic, peeled and minced
1 yellow onion, peeled and chopped
4 cups vegetable stock
2 cups raw pumpkin, peeled, seeded, and diced
1/2 cup quinoa
1/4 teaspoon salt
1/4 cup almond butter
2 cups kale, chopped
1 tablespoon tamari

1 tablespoon honey
1 tablespoon freshly grated ginger root
2 tablespoon fresh-squeezed lemon juice

Directions:

- Soak the beans overnight in enough water to cover. Drain and set aside.

- In a large dutch oven, melt the coconut oil and stir in the garlic and onion. Sauté until the onion becomes translucent.

- Add the vegetable stock, pumpkin, drained beans, quinoa and the salt. Simmer with a lid on for 45 minutes.

- Place the almond butter in a small bowl and add a half cup of the stew liquid, stirring to make a paste. Stir this into the stew.

- Add the kale and cook 5 more minutes.

- Remove from the heat and stir in the tamari, honey, ginger and lemon juice.

Yield: 4 servings

BLACK FRIED RICE

The purple-black color of black rice indicates that it is full of powerful antioxidants. This recipe is full of delicious flavor.

Ingredients:

2 tablespoons coconut oil
1 small yellow onion, peeled and diced
1 bunch scallions, sliced with the white parts separated from the green
2 medium carrots, peeled and diced

2 cloves garlic, minced
1 tablespoon fresh grated ginger root
1 cup snap peas, sliced
3 cups cooked black rice (pre-cook 1 cup of dry rice)
1 tablespoon tamari
1 teaspoon sriracha
2 teaspoons sesame oil
2 beaten eggs
1 tablespoon hemp seed

Directions:

- Use a wok or nonstick skillet and heat up the coconut oil.

- Sauté the onion, white scallions, and carrot over high heat until they become soft and start to turn brown. This will take about 5 minutes.

- Add the garlic, ginger, peas and green scallions and stir-fry about 2 minutes.

- Fold in the cooked rice.

- In a bowl, combine the tamari, sriracha, and sesame oil. Pour this mixture over the rice and stir to coat.

- Push the rice around the edges of the pan to make a hole in the center. Whisk the eggs in a small bowl and pour in the middle, stirring gently until almost set.

- Pour the hemp seed on top of the egg and start mixing with a fork to incorporate the rice with the egg mixture.

- Serve in bowls and enjoy.

Yield: 4 servings

This chapter has armed you with an arsenal of hearty dinner recipes, all anti-inflammatory in nature. You should eat well for weeks! Now, let's turn to lighter fare, snack foods so delicious you wouldn't guess they were healthy, too.

Chapter 9: Sweet and Savory Anti-Inflammatory Snacks

Just because you have chronic inflammation, there's no reason to forego the good stuff! This chapter gives you recipes for mouthwatering pie and cookies, along with tasty chips and dips.

KALE CHIPS

Kale can be baked into delicious crispy chips that even the kids will love.

Ingredients:

2 bunches of curly sage with stems removed, washed and torn into bite sized pieces
1 cup grated sweet potato
1 cup cashews, soaked and softened in water about 2 hours
2 tablespoons nutritional yeast (found at health food stores)
The juice of 1 lemon
2 tablespoons honey
1/2 teaspoon sea salt
2 tablespoons water

Directions:

- Put the kale in a large bowl and set aside.

- In a blender or food processor, process the sweet potato, softened cashews yeast, lemon juice, honey, salt and water until smooth. Pour this mixture over the kale and toss with your hands to coat the leaves.

- Spread the kale leaves out on a large cookie sheet in a single layer without touching.

- Turn on the oven to its lowest setting.

- Prop the oven door slightly ajar and dehydrate the chips for about 2 hours, turning the cookie sheet and watching to make sure the chips do not burn.

- When crisp, remove from the oven and let cool. Store in an airtight container.

Yield: about 8 cups of chips.

BRUSSEL SPROUT CHIPS

Yes, you can make chips from brussel sprouts. You will need to use only the loose outer leaves of about 2 pounds of sprouts. Use the rest in other recipes.

Ingredients:

2 cups brussels sprout leaves
2 tablespoons ghee
Kosher salt
Lemon zest

Directions:

- Preheat your oven to 350 degrees Fahrenheit and cover two cookie sheets with parchment paper.

- Place the leaves in a large bowl and pour melted ghee over top and add salt.

- Bake for 8 to 10 minutes or until the leaves are crispy. If they are soft at all, put them back in the oven.

- While still hot, sprinkle the lemon zest over the leaves. Serve warm.

Yield: 4 servings

MUSHROOM CHIPS

King oyster mushrooms work best for this dish because they are firm, large, and have an earthy flavor.

Ingredients:

16 ounces of king oyster mushrooms
2 tablespoons ghee
Kosher salt and ground pepper to taste

Directions:

- Preheat the oven to 300 degrees Fahrenheit and line two cookie sheets with parchment paper.

- Cut each mushroom in half lengthwise, then cut with a mandolin into 1/8 inch slices or strips. Place them on cookie sheets with some room in between. Melt the ghee and brush it over the mushrooms, then season with the salt and pepper.

- Bake for 45 minutes to 1 hour, until they are completely crisp. Store in airtight containers.

Yield: 2 to 4 servings

HUMMUS WITH CELERY

Hummus is delicious as a dip or spread. The garlic and turmeric only add to the healthfulness. In this recipe, you fill the indentation of celery with hummus and it makes a lovely treat. You can also sprinkle sunflower seeds atop the hummus in place of paprika.

Ingredients:

1/4 cup lemon juice
1/4 cup tahini
3 cloves of garlic, crushed

2 tablespoons extra virgin olive oil
1/2 teaspoon salt
1/2 teaspoon cumin
1 (15–ounce) can chickpeas
2 to 3 tablespoons water
Dash of paprika
6 stalks celery, cut into 2-inch pieces
3 tablespoons salsa

Directions:

- Use a food processor or blender to mix the lemon juice and tahini for about a minute, until it is smooth. Scrape the sides down and process for 30 more seconds.

- Add the garlic, olive oil, salt, and cumin. Blend for about 1 minute.

- Drain the chickpeas, add half of them to the food processor, and blend for another minute. Scrape down the sides, add the other half of the chickpeas, and process until smooth, about 2 minutes. If it seems a little too thick, add water, 1 tablespoon at a time until you reach the desired consistency.

- Fill the celery sticks with hummus and sprinkle paprika on top.

- Serve with salsa for dipping.

Yield: about 4 servings

HUMMUS DEVILED EGGS

The yolk is not used for these eggs, but save it to use in other recipes. This is a wonderful anti-inflammatory protein-boosting snack.

Ingredients:

6 hard-boiled eggs
1/2 cup hummus
Paprika

Directions:

Slice the hardboiled eggs in half lengthwise and remove the yolk.

Fill the egg whites with hummus and sprinkle with paprika before serving.

Yield: 6 servings (12 deviled eggs)

CAULIFLOWER SNACK

This recipe is great for snacking on during a movie or television show and it is easy to make. Just don't crunch it too loudly to hear!

Ingredients:

1 head of cauliflower
4 tablespoons extra virgin olive oil
1 teaspoon salt

Directions:

- Preheat your oven to 425 degrees Fahrenheit and prepare two cookie sheets by lining them with parchment paper.

- Trim off the cauliflower florets and discard the core. Cut the florets into golf-ball-sized pieces.

- Place the cauliflower in a bowl, and pour olive oil over them and sprinkle with salt. Mix to coat. Spread in a single layer, not touching.

- Roast about 1 hour, turning the cauliflower three to four times until golden brown. Serve warm.

Yield: 4 servings

MANDARIN COTTAGE CHEESE

Cottage cheese is a dairy product, but it contains a slow-digesting protein that makes it a favorite of athletes. The low-fat variety will help with cholesterol management. This recipe includes a touch of healthy sweetness and adds a slight crunch to the mix. Enjoy!

Ingredients:

1/2 cup low-fat cottage cheese
1/2 cup canned mandarin oranges
1 1/2 tablespoons slivered almonds

Directions:

- Place the cottage cheese in a bowl.
- Drain the mandarin oranges, place them atop the cottage cheese, and sprinkle with almonds.

Yield: 1 serving

CUCUMBER YOGURT

If you like cucumbers, you will love this snack. The added cashews provide a satisfying crunch to offset the soft yogurt.

Ingredients:

1 cup cucumbers, skin removed and chopped in chunks
2 tablespoons chopped cashews
1/4 cup fat-free Greek yogurt
2 teaspoons fresh-squeezed lemon juice

1 teaspoon fresh dill, chopped fine

Directions:

- Peel and chop the cucumbers, then place them in a bowl.
- Add the cashews, yogurt, lemon juice, and dill.
- Mix well, grab a spoon, and enjoy.

Yield: 1 serving

ANTI-INFLAMMATORY KEY LIME PIE

This recipe is gluten- and sugar-free, but dates and honey give it a delightful sweetness alongside the lime's tart flavor.

Ingredients:

1 cup walnuts
1 cup unsweetened shredded coconut
1/4 teaspoon sea salt
1/2 cup pitted and chopped medjool dates
3 firm avocados
1/2 cup honey
3 tablespoons lime juice
1 teaspoon lime zest
Pinch of sea salt
Lime slices

Directions:

- In a food processor, combine the walnuts, coconut, and the salt, then process until coarsely ground.
- Add the dates and process until the mixture looks like bread crumbs, trying to clump together.

- Press the mixture into the bottom and sides of a non-stick greased 9-inch pie pan. Use your fingers or the back of a spoon to press the crust into an even layer. Put the crust into the freezer for 15 minutes while preparing the filling.

- Use the food processor again and combine the avocado, honey, lime juice, lime zest, and salt. Process until smooth.

- Pour the filling into the now-chilled piecrust and place it in the refrigerator for 20 minutes.

- Garnish with fresh lime slices and serve cold. Store any leftovers in the refrigerator.

Yield: 8 servings

STRAWBERRY-ALMOND FRUIT POPS

Here is another yogurt treat, surprisingly delicious and delightfully cooling on a hot day.

Ingredients:

1 1/2 tablespoons almonds
1 cup strawberries
3 cups plain low-fat yogurt
6 paper cups
6 popsicle sticks

Directions:

- Place the almonds and strawberries in a food processor and blend until chunky.

- Add the yogurt and pulse 3 to 4 times.

- Divide the mixture between 6 small paper cups and place a clean popsicle stick in the middle.

- Freeze overnight. Peel the cups off before eating.

Yield: 6 fruitpops.

BERRY-NUT YOGURT

This is a yogurt and blueberry snack, super easy to make and enjoy.

Ingredients:

1/3 cup fresh blueberries
1/4 cup fat-free Greek yogurt
1 tablespoon slivered almonds

Directions:

- Mix the blueberries and yogurt in a bowl.

- Sprinkle with almonds, grab a spoon, and dig in!

Yield: 1 serving

PROTEASE-FREE JELLED FRUIT

Quick nutritional note: Proteases, also known as proteolytic enzymes or peptidases, are a type of enzyme you normally *want* to include in your diet, because they help to regulate your immune response. However, they do their job so well that your gelatin just won't gel in their presence. Fruits containing protease include fresh pineapple (you can use canned, because the canning process destroys the proteases), kiwi, mango, guava, papaya, and fig. The protease can be deactivated by steaming these fruits for five minutes before adding to gelatin

This recipe is a gelatin treat with lots of fruit and walnuts. You can leave the nuts out altogether or substitute almonds or cashews if you prefer. You can also use any fruits you desire. The flavor extracts are what really make the flavor pop.

Ingredients:

2 cups water
4 envelopes unflavored gelatin
3/4 cup fresh raspberries
1/4 cup seedless red or green grapes
1 kiwi, peeled and sliced
1 cup strawberries, diced
1 tablespoon orange extract
1/2 teaspoon strawberry extract
1 tablespoon banana extract
2 tablespoons walnuts
Mint leaves

Directions:

- Steam the kiwi for 5 minutes to break down the protease.

- Place 2 cups of water in a saucepan over high heat and sprinkle in the gelatin. Stir until the gelatin dissolves. Remove from the heat.

- Stir in the fruit and both extracts.

- Pour into an 8-inch square pan and let it cool to room temperature.

- Once cool, add the nuts. Place in the refrigerator until set.

- Cut into fourths, place on dessert plates, and garnish with mint.

Yield: 4 servings

TOFU PUDDING

This is a nutty, fruity pudding made from tofu, fruit, and almonds. The protein powder can be found in any health food store.

Ingredients:

12 ounces silken tofu, softened and well drained
2 scoops of protein powder
3/4 cup blueberries
1 cup strawberries
1 teaspoon honey
1 teaspoon pumpkin pie spice
1 teaspoon vanilla
4 almonds
Fresh mint leaves

Directions:

- Blend the tofu and protein powder in a blender until well mixed.

- Add the blueberries, strawberries, honey, pumpkin pie spice, and vanilla. Blend until smooth.

- Cover and chill for at least two hours.

- Spoon into four dessert bowls and top with an almond and a mint leaf before serving.

Yield: 4 servings

SPICY BAKED APPLES

Baked apples is a classic recipe, chock full of flavor. This version uses honey and apple juice as healthy, natural sweeteners. Use a tart, firm apple like MacIntosh or Jonathan.

Ingredients:

2 large dates, pitted and chopped

1/2 cups nuts of choice or sunflower seeds, diced
1/4 cup dried cranberries
1 teaspoon grated ginger root
1/4 teaspoon ground nutmeg
1 teaspoon ground cinnamon
1/4 teaspoon ground cloves
4 apples
1/4 cup honey
1 cup unsweetened apple juice

Directions:

- Preheat the oven to 325 degrees and grease an 8-inch square pan. I prefer to use coconut oil.

- In a bowl, combine the dates, nuts, cranberries, ginger, nutmeg, cinnamon and cloves. Set aside

- Leave the peels on the apples and cut out the core. Stuff the center of the apple with the date-nut combination.

- Place the stuffed apples in the prepared pan and drizzle with honey. Pour apple juice in the bottom of the pan and bake for 30 to 35 minutes or until the apples become soft. Serve warm.

Yield: 4 servings

APPLE CRISP

This is another classic recipe, with healthy coconut and rolled oats. It uses almond meal as an anti-inflammatory alternative to flour. Melt the coconut oil by placing it in a glass dish and setting it in a larger container of hot water.

Ingredients:

Topping:
1 1/2 cups old-fashioned rolled oats

2/3 cup shredded, unsweetened coconut
1 teaspoon salt
1/2 cup stevia
1/3 cup almond meal
1/4 teaspoon ground nutmeg
2 teaspoons ground cinnamon
1 cup nuts, coarsely chopped
3 tablespoon melted coconut oil.

Apple filling:
10 tart apples
1/2 cup stevia
2 tablespoons fresh-squeezed lemon juice
1 tablespoon ground cinnamon
1/4 cup arrowroot flour
1/4 teaspoon salt
3 tablespoons melted coconut oil
1 teaspoon vanilla
The zest of 1 orange

Directions:

- Preheat the oven to 350 degrees, Fahrenheit and grease a 9 by 13-inch baking pan with coconut oil.

- Mix the topping ingredients in a bowl and set aside.

- Mix the filling ingredients (except for the apples) in a second large bowl.

- Leave the skins on the apples, if desired. Core them and slice very thin (1/8 inch thick).

- Toss the apples in the filling ingredients to coat evenly. Place the apple mixture in a baking pan and spread the topping over it all, pressing down firmly.

- Place in the oven with a pan underneath to catch any drips.

- Bake for 25 minutes or until the topping is brown and juices are bubbling. Apples should be soft.

- Cool slightly on a rack and serve warm.

Yield: 6 to 8 servings

APPLESAUCE TREAT

If you like both applesauce and cottage cheese, you'll love this combination!

Ingredients:

1/4 cup low fat cottage cheese
1/4 cup unsweetened applesauce
1/2 teaspoon cinnamon
1 1/2 teaspoons toasted slivered almonds

Directions:

- Mix the cottage cheese and applesauce in a bowl, stirring well.

- Sprinkle with cinnamon and mix well.

- Sprinkle the top with almonds, pick up your spoon and enjoy.

Yield: 1 serving

BROWNIES AVOCADO

Avocados are great anti-inflammatory food. This recipe uses some unusual ingredients for brownies but it sure tastes good.

Ingredients:

1/2 cup almond meal
3/4 cup cocoa powder
1 1/2 teaspoon instant coffee (with or without caffeine, as you wish)
2 teaspoons ground cinnamon
1/2 teaspoon salt
2 cups nuts or seeds, chopped
1 avocado
1 apple, cored and chopped, with the skin on
1 cup cooked and diced sweet potato
4 tablespoons ground chia seeds
1 teaspoon vanilla
1/2 cup almond butter
1/2 cup coconut butter, softened
1/4 cup coconut oil
2 1/4 cup stevia

Directions:

- Preheat oven to 350 degrees Fahrenheit and line a 9 by 13-inch pan with parchment. Let it overlap the sides to make handles for lifting the brownies out when done.

- In a bowl combine the almond meal, cocoa, coffee, cinnamon, salt and nuts. Whisk and set aside.

- Place the remaining ingredients in a food processor and mix until smooth. Add the ingredients in the bowl and pulse. This combination should be chunky.

- Pour into prepared pan and bake for 25 minutes.

- Let cool and chill in the refrigerator for two hours before slicing. The baked product will be a little gooey, so refrigerating it makes the brownies easier to cut. The chilled results will be somewhat crumbly.

Yield: 6 to 8 servings

LEMONY GINGER COOKIES

Yes, you can have cookies on an anti-inflammatory diet. I've just replaced the bad stuff with anti-inflammatory ingredients. These cookies have a fresh lemon flavor with the zing of ginger. The nutritional yeast, found at health food stores gives the cookie a bit of a buttery taste.

Ingredients:

1/2 cup arrowroot flour
1 1/2 cups stevia
3/4 teaspoon salt
1/2 teaspoon baking soda
1 teaspoon nutritional yeast
3 inches of ginger root, peeled and diced
1 1/2 cup coconut butter, softened
Zest of 1 lemon
2 teaspoons vanilla

Directions:

- Preheat the oven to 350 degrees and line two or three cookie sheets with parchment paper.

- Mix the arrowroot flour, stevia, salt, soda, and yeast in a bowl.

- In another bowl combine the remaining ingredients and mix well.

- Add in the dry ingredients gradually until well combined. If the dough is too soft, add another 1 to 2 tablespoons of arrowroot powder. The dough will stiffen when chilled, so be careful.

- Wrap the dough in a piece of parchment and press it flat. Chill for 30 minutes.

- Take a chunk of the chilled dough and flatten it between two pieces of parchment until it is 1/8 inch thick. Dust with a little arrowroot powder and cut into shapes.

- Place on baking sheets about 1 inch apart and bake 10 to 12 minutes. Cool on cookie sheets for 15 minutes before removing.

Yield: 2 1/2 dozen cookies

PUMPKIN CHOCOLATE CHIP COOKIES

This recipe calls for pumpkin, cooked and drained (you can use canned pumpkin), almond flour and arrowroot flour. It does call for nuts, but they are optional.

Ingredients:

3 tablespoons arrowroot flour
1 cup almond meal
1 tablespoon pumpkin pie spice
1/2 teaspoon salt
1/2 cup pumpkin, cooked and drained (option: use canned pumpkin)
2 large eggs
1 tablespoon vanilla
1/2 teaspoon maple flavoring
2 cups stevia or 1 1/2 cups honey
1 cup coconut butter
1 1/2 cups chopped nuts
1 cup dark chocolate chips

Directions:

- Preheat the oven to 350 degrees Fahrenheit. and line 2 cookie sheets with parchment paper.

- In a bowl combine the arrowroot flour, almond meal, spice, and salt. Mix well.

- In a mixer bowl, combine the pumpkin and eggs and beat well. Add the vanilla and flavoring and mix together.

- Add in the stevia or honey and the coconut butter; mix well.

- Add the dry ingredients to the wet, gradually, until well combined. Stir in the nuts and chocolate chips by hand.

- Put the dough in the refrigerator to firm up, about 15 minutes.

- Roll the dough by tablespoonful into balls and set them one inch apart on the baking sheets. Slightly flatten with fingers.

- Bake 18 to 20 minutes or until just brown on edges. Cool on cookie sheets and remove when cool.

TOASTED PUMPKIN SEEDS

If you used real pumpkin in the last recipe, save the seeds, wash them well, and let them dry for a day or so.

Ingredients:

1 to 2 cups pumpkin seeds
Water
1 teaspoon salt
1/2 teaspoon extra virgin olive oil
Sea salt

Directions:

- Put seeds in a saucepan and cover with water. Add salt.

- Bring it to a boil and boil for 10 minutes.

- Simmer uncovered for 10 more minutes. This makes the seeds very crispy when baked. Drain the seeds and pat dry with a paper towel.

- Cover a baking sheet with parchment paper and spread out the seeds in a single layer.

- Sprinkle with salt and bake in a preheated 325 degree Fahrenheit oven for 10 minutes, stirring half way through.

Cool, then store in an airtight container.

I hope you're enjoying these healthy sweet and savory treats. There are more treats ahead.

Chapter 10: Spectacular Anti-Inflammatory Smoothies and Juices

Smoothies make a great start to the day and a wonderful pick-me-up treat in the afternoon. Although some juices are not suitable for an anti-inflammatory diet, there are a few that you may find beneficial. The protein powder included in some of these recipes gives your drink a little extra punch of protein; It can easily turn use it as a smoothie meal. Protein powder is found in your local health food store.

Here are some smoothie and juice recipes just about anyone in the family will enjoy. Each recipe makes a single serving unless otherwise indicated.

MERRY BERRY SMOOTHIE

Use one or more of your favorite fresh berries to make this smoothie. It will give a nice burst of calm energy.

Ingredients:

2 or more ice cubes, depending on how thick you want your smoothie
4 teaspoons tahini
1 1/2 cups berries
3 scoops protein powder

Directions:

- Mix all the ingredients in a blender for about one minute or until smooth and creamy.

- Pour into a glass and enjoy.

CHOCO-BLUEBERRY SMOOTHIE

Blueberries and chocolate are delicious together; you can use frozen blueberries or even strawberries, if you prefer.

Ingredients:

2/3 cups frozen blueberries
3/4 cup almond milk
2 teaspoons honey
1 tablespoon almond butter
2 teaspoons cocoa powder
2 scoops protein powder
2 or more ice cubes, depending on your preferred consistency

Directions:

- Toss all ingredients in a blender and blend until smooth.

- If it is too thick, add another ice cube.

ANTI-INFLAMMATORY **MINT JULEP**

Mint and strawberry taste great together. You use green tea in this recipe, brewed and cooled. green tea is an antioxidant. This isn't really a smoothie, but a nice thick drink that is totally refreshing.

Ingredients:

1 cup green tea
2 large apples, juiced
1/4 lemon, juiced
1.1/2 cups whole strawberries, juiced
12 peppermint leaves, juiced or 5 drops peppermint extract
3/4 cup honey (taste first, you might not need this much)

Directions:

- Brew the tea and let it cool.

- Juice the fruit with the peppermint leaves.

- Pour the cooled tea into the juice.

- Stir in the honey and pour over ice.

LIMEY RASPBERRY SMOOTHIE

Talk about refreshing! This smoothie will satisfy any thirst and almost any hunger. You get a great protein boost from the yogurt and almonds, so there's no protein powder needed.

Ingredients:

1/2 cup fat-free Greek yogurt
1 cup almond milk or soy milk
1 cup fresh or frozen raspberries
Juice of 1 lime
3 tablespoons slivered almonds

Directions:
- Blend all ingredients well in a blender.

- Add ice if too thick.

- Pour into a chilled glass and enjoy!

PAPAYA SMOOTHIE

The tropical flavor of papaya is delicious; papaya contains an enzyme that helps your stomach digest protein. This recipe also contains flaxseed oil, which helps to prevent and heal inflammation in the bones and joints.

Ingredients:

2 cups chopped papaya
3/4 cup chopped mango
2 teaspoons fresh-squeezed lemon juice

1 cup almond milk
1 teaspoon flaxseed oil
1/4 teaspoon vanilla
2 teaspoons minced fresh gingerroot
1/4 teaspoon ground cinnamon
5 drops liquid stevia
1/4 teaspoon lemon zest
1 cup ice cubes

Directions:

- Blend all ingredients on high until smooth and creamy.

- Pour into two glasses and enjoy.

Yield: 2 servings

TROPICAL PUNCH SMOOTHIE

Get all the flavor of the tropics in this delicious smoothie, with its full complement of mango, pineapple, peaches, lime, and coconut. You can use either fresh or frozen fruit for this recipe. The included curry and pepper flakes just give the smoothie some pizzazz; they don't make it hot.

Ingredients:

1 cup diced peaches
1 cup diced pineapple
1 cup diced mango
1/2 teaspoon lime zest
3/4 cups canned coconut milk, shaken
2 cups ice cubes (use only with fresh fruit. Use ice sparingly with frozen fruit)
1/4 teaspoon yellow curry powder
A few red pepper flakes
1 pinch salt
1 tablespoon honey (optional)

Directions:

- Blend all ingredients on high until smooth and creamy.
- Taste first before adding honey; it might be sweet enough already.

Yield: 2 smoothies.

PINEAPPLE SALSA SMOOTHIE

Pineapple is good for the digestive system; it also relieves stomach cramps and helps to keep your white blood cells calm. The combination of pineapple, spinach, cucumber, and onion may sound strange, but it's actually quite delicious. Just give it a try.

Ingredients:

2 1/2 cups diced pineapple
1 cup baby spinach, packed
2 tablespoons cucumber, peeled and chopped
1 1/2 teaspoon red onion, finely chopped
2 tablespoons fresh-squeezed lime juice
1 pinch lime zest
1/4 cup cilantro, finely chopped
1 teaspoon jalapeno, seeded and finely chopped
1 cup ice cubes (omit if using frozen pineapple)
1 tablespoon honey

Directions:

- Mix all ingredients in a blender until creamy.
- Serve in a chilled glass.

Yield: 2 servings

TROPICAL THREE-P JUICE

The three Ps are peaches, pineapple, and pear. This cooling beverage is most effective on a hot summer day, but you can enjoy its anti-inflammatory properties any day of the year.

Ingredients:

1/2 pineapple, juiced
1 medium pear, juiced
1 large peach, pitted and juiced

Directions:

- Process all ingredients and mix well.

- Serve over ice.

INDIA-INSPIRED CARROT SMOOTHIE

This smoothie boasts a bunch of delicious antioxidant ingredients, including turmeric and ginger.

Ingredients:

2 cups carrots (yield: 1/2 cup fresh carrot juice)
1 1/2 cups water
1 cup frozen or fresh pineapple
1 ripe banana, peeled, sliced and frozen.
1/2 tablespoon fresh grated ginger root
1/4 cup turmeric
1 tablespoon fresh-squeezed lemon juice
1 cup almond milk

Directions:

- Juice the carrots by adding the water and carrots to a high-speed blender. Blend until smooth. Add more water if it is too thick.

- Place a large square of cheesecloth over a bowl and set the carrot mixture in the center. Bring up the edges to enclose the carrot mixture and squeeze out the juice. Set aside the carrot solids to use in carrot muffins or other baking dishes.

- Set the juice aside.

- Blend the rest of the ingredients.

- Add the carrot juice, mixing well, and serve.

Yield: 2 servings

FRUITY KALE SMOOTHIE

Kale, avocado, berries, and banana make for a great start to your morning!

Ingredients:

1 1/2 cups cold water, or 1 cup water and several ice cubes for thicker consistency
4 cups kale, chopped, with ribs cut out
1 banana chunked
1/2 avocado, chopped
3/4 cup frozen blueberries
2 tablespoons protein powder
1 teaspoon extra virgin olive oil

Directions:

- Blend the water and kale first and add the banana and avocado.

- Add the berries and powder until smooth and creamy.

- Drizzle in the olive oil and pulse to mix in.

Yield: 2 servings

FRUIT-VEGGIE MISHMASH JUICE

This juice has a wild mix of fruits and vegetables, but the flavor is unusually good.

Ingredients:

2 large red cabbage leaves
3 medium-sized carrots
1 (8-inch-long) cucumber
1 peeled mango
1/2 cup whole strawberries
2 medium apples

Directions:

- Process all the ingredients in a juicer.//
- Serve over ice.

NATURALLY RED JUICE

This juice has a lovely natural red tinge and a delicious flavor. No food coloring added; the cabbage takes care of that.

Ingredients:

2 medium pears
4 leaves of red cabbage
1/2 lemon with rind on

Directions:

- Process all ingredients in a juicer.
- Serve over ice.

GINGERY JUICE

This drink contains a mixture fruits and vegetables. They actually taste pretty good together and the freshly grated ginger adds some eye-popping flavor.

Ingredients:

5 medium carrots
1 (8-inch-long) cucumber
2 handfuls of baby spinach
1 medium pear
1 medium apple
1 whole lemon, with rind

Directions:

- Juice all ingredients together.

- Serve over ice.

PEACHY KEEN SMOOTHIE

This recipe uses peaches, but for variety you can substitute 3 or 4 apricots.

Ingredients:

2 teaspoons almond butter
2 tablespoons almond milk
2 scoops protein powder
2 peaches, pitted, with skin left on
1 sprig of mint

Directions:

- Combine all ingredients, except mint, in a blender and blend.

- Add a little ice if too thick.

- Pour into a glass and garnish with mint.

PARSLEY AND GRAPE LEMONADE SMOOTHIE

Use green or red grapes for this delicious, thirst-quenching drink. Just make sure they are seedless.

Ingredients:

1/2 small avocado, peeled and pitted
3 cups seedless grapes
1 bunch flat-leaf parsley, chopped
1/2 cup fresh-squeezed lemon juice
2 teaspoons grated ginger root
5 drops liquid stevia
2 cups ice cubes

Directions:

- Blend all ingredients until smooth.

- Pour in a glass and enjoy.

HEALTHY BANANA MACA SMOOTHIE

Maca powder is made from the root of a Peruvian plant; the powder is available in health food stores. It is chock-full of amino acids, iron, and manganese that give your muscles an energy boost. No ice is needed, because frozen banana provides the chill.

Ingredients:

3 medium bananas, sliced and frozen
2 cups coconut water
1 cup baby spinach, loosely packed
1 tablespoon chia seeds

1 teaspoon maca powder
1/4 cup ground cinnamon

Directions:

- Blend all ingredients until creamy.

- Pour into a chilled glass and serve.

AUTUMN SPICE JUICE

The flavors of these ingredients mingle to give you the taste of Fall in a glass.

Ingredients:

1 medium apple (use a firm apple like Braeburn, Fuji, or McIntosh)
2 slices of canned pineapple rings, drained
1 (1-inch) thumb of ginger root, peeled
1 golden beet
1/2 lemon
1/4 teaspoon pumpkin pie spice

Directions:

- Process in juicer.

- Shake well and serve immediately.

FOURTH OF JULY JUICE

We call it Fourth of July juice because we had strawberries, watermelon and peaches in the house and mixed them all together for a treat one year on the Fourth. The name stuck and it became a Fourth of July tradition.

Ingredients:

2 cups diced watermelon (use seedless watermelon or remove the seeds)
1 cup whole strawberries
1 medium peach, pitted without removing skin
1/2 lime
7 mint leaves

Directions:

- Process all ingredients in a juicer.

- Serve over ice.

PINK POMEGRANATE JUICE

Pomegranates are known for their health benefits. They are an antioxidant and taste delicious. The best thing about juicing is you don't have to remove the seeds; you just peel it, break it up, and pop it in the juicer.

Ingredients:

1 (4-inch diameter) pomegranate
1 large apple
1 large orange
1/2 lemon
1 inch piece of gingerroot, peeled

Directions:

- Process all ingredients in the juicer.

- Stir and serve over ice.

HOLIDAY PUMPKIN JUICE

You don't have to serve this juice on Thanksgiving, but your guests will love you if you do.

Ingredients:

2 cups of cubed pumpkin
2 medium apples
1 cup fresh cranberries
1 orange, peeled
1 inch of peeled ginger root
1/4 teaspoon nutmeg
1 teaspoon cinnamon

Directions:

- Process all ingredients except the nutmeg and cinnamon in the juicer.

- Mix in the spices and serve.

Yield: 2 servings

Conclusion

I hope this book was able to help you understand chronic inflammation and give you the tools you need in order to combat it successfully.

The next step is to start swapping out "bad" foods for good ones. These ideas should get you started:

- Pick a bad food you're willing to give up, then choose a good food you aren't eating on a regular basis as its replacement.

- Clear out your refrigerator and cupboards of the bad food item.

- Attach a note to your shopping list to remind you to avoid your targeted bad food and focus on using the new good food.

- Look at the recipes in this book to get ideas how you can start incorporating that good food into your diet. Many of the beneficial spices can be worked into your existing foods, to add flavor as well as anti-inflammatory effects, so feel free to experiment with new taste combinations.

- Purchase your good food and choose to use it in several dishes over the next few weeks.

Use this same process when it comes to including vitamins, minerals, and other supplements into your lifestyle. Don't shock your body with too many changes all at once, but introduce new substances one or two at a time.

You are venturing on a path that can only bring greater health and energy to your mind and body. It's important that you give yourself the time you need to adjust to a new food choice before making another adjustment to your eating habits. Let your mind and body recover at their own pace.

At the same time, watch for changes in your energy levels, in your levels of pain, and in your digestion. To facilitate this process, drink plenty of water; it will help your body flush out unwanted toxins, and your body will benefit from adequate hydration.

Over time you will grow in body awareness. You will become more aware of your energy levels and will notice the impact that different foods and supplements have on your physical well-being.

Of course, many of these changes will occur, not immediately, but over time, so let yourself rest patiently in the process and know that you are doing yourself an incredible amount of good each day as you pursue a healthy lifestyle. Remind yourself that every small change to your diet will have amplified positive results in the long run. Over time, these choices will add up to greater health, a balanced immune system, fewer episodes of inflammation, and the ability to experience all the good life has to offer.

Thanks for reading.

If this book helped you or someone you know in any way, then please spare a few moments right now to leave a nice review.

My Other Books

Be sure to check out my author page at: https://www.amazon.com/author/susanhollister

UK: http://amzn.to/2qiEzA9

Or simply type my name into the search bar: Susan Hollister

Thank You